Solving the Pain Puzzle

Solving the Pain Puzzle

Cases from 25 Years as a Physical Therapist

RICK OLDERMAN, MSPT

Foreword by ELIZABETH SEBESTYEN, M.D.

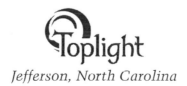

Toplight
Jefferson, North Carolina

Library of Congress and British Library
Cataloguing data are available

ISBN (print) 978-1-4766-9069-8 ∞
ISBN (ebook) 978-1-4766-4862-0

Front cover images: © design36/Video Render/Inkoly/Shutterstock

Printed in the United States of America

Toplight is an imprint of McFarland & Company, Inc., Publishers

*Box 611, Jefferson, North Carolina 28640
www.toplightbooks.com*

For Mom, who asked for more stories

Acknowledgments

None of the stories in this book could have been written without the dedication of previous health professionals in uncovering the secrets behind how we are and how we function. My journey began with Dr. Shirley Sahrmann PT, PhD, FAPTA, whose textbooks, seminars and research provided me the foundation from which to help patients with difficult pain but also explore others' approaches as well. Thomas Myers' contribution to understanding fascial patterns has also been instrumental in my exploration of distant connections in our bodies. Lastly Thomas Hanna PhD and Eleanor Criswell EdD, C-IAYT, who together created the Hanna Somatics training, deserve my deepest thanks for developing their unique and powerful approach to solving pain.

Additionally I owe a debt of gratitude to Dr. Noah Charney whose advice helped make this book more readable.

I would also like to thank my medical illustrators, Martin Huber and Meghan M. Shoemaker, whose images help my readers see key relationships featured in *Solving the Pain Puzzle*.

Table of Contents

Foreword
by Elizabeth Sebestyen, M.D.

"Your pain is *not* incurable. It is caused by how you use your body. I'll help you identify and correct poor movement habits to end your pain. Even if nothing else has worked for you." This is the motto accompanying Rick Olderman's professional logo. And he holds true to his promise, whether your pain was caused by a recent injury or surgery or has been nagging you for years!

Over the next pages you will meet some of his patients and learn about their incredible recoveries. You will read about Rick's victories in unlocking contracted muscles and healing migraines, neck pain, shoulder pain and much more. Most importantly you will get to know Rick as he genuinely shares the ups and downs of his journey with all its frustrations and self-doubts. These hurdles are not uncommon in the life of a healthcare professional and can make or break him or her. They pushed Rick almost to the brink, only to make him the best physical therapist I had the pleasure to work with. They pushed him to find answers to the *whys*—the root cause of the problems; they pushed him back to the anatomy lab, to study nonconventional approaches and work out holistic solutions that are sometimes deceivingly simple.

My own story was not unique enough to make it to this book, and I am thankful for that. In medicine you never want to be an interesting case! Perhaps it was not unusual for Rick to help someone walk pain free after a complex ankle fracture and three surgeries. For me it was huge! And not only did I walk, but I was even able to handle the hilly, cobblestoned streets of Portugal shortly after my surgeon allowed me to walk!

1

Foreword by Elizabeth Sebestyen, M.D.

Without pain!

Rick helped me tremendously and I referred many of my patients, friends and family members to him.

Elizabeth Sebestyen, M.D., is an internal medicine physician integrating medical acupuncture into a busy primary care practice. She has always appreciated Rick Olderman's holistic approach and the lasting pain relief that his techniques and exercises offered to patients.

Preface

I've been interested in solving pain since I became a physical therapist in 1996. The problem I immediately ran into at my first job was that I clearly hadn't acquired the tools to do this. Over the years, as I unraveled how the body creates and solves chronic musculoskeletal pain, describing my emerging approach left me scratching my head. Only recently have I found the words to succinctly express how *I* solve pain, as distinguished from how I was *taught* to solve pain.

I describe it as a systems approach, as opposed to a component approach.

Through physical therapy school and today, evidence-based treatment has been the buzz phrase to describe how we should help others heal their bodies. Everything we do must have medical evidence to support it. To create evidence, it seems, we study and report on small pieces of our body puzzle—components. While this is an important process to unravel how we tick, this rule severely constrains creative thinking and the observation necessary to solve difficult cases. Had I restricted my treatment philosophy to only what was supported by medical evidence, none of the stories you're about to read would have had happy endings. At some point, we need to understand how to put the pieces of our puzzle back together to make Humpty Dumpty whole again—to help him function as a system (as much as a walking egg who chooses to sit on a wall can work as a system).

So, while evidence is important, synthesizing that information (adding a pinch of extrapolation here and of creativity there) to form concrete solutions becomes meaningful—especially to those who are suffering with chronic pain.

This book represents my efforts to create an evidence-directed, yet more holistic, approach to solving our body's pain puzzles.

Introduction

I would become Sherlock Holmes.

I'm probably not the first child to have concocted this master plan, but I'm likely among the few who actually made it happen. I solve mysteries. Not the kind involving butlers in the study with the candelabra.

They do, however, involve bodies.

⊐⊏ ⊐⊏ ⊐⊏

Let us consider the case of the Boscombe Valley Mystery, penned by Sir Arthur Conan Doyle, one of 58 short stories (as well as four novels) starring his famous character, Sherlock Holmes. After examining the site of a murder by bludgeoning in a forest, Holmes and Police Inspector Lestrade discuss the crime scene. Holmes hands Lestrade a rock.

"This may interest you, Lestrade," he remarked, holding it out. "The murder was done with it."

"I see no marks."

"There are none."

"How do you know, then?"

"The grass was growing under it. It had only lain there a few days. There was no sign of a place whence it had been taken. It corresponds with the injuries. There is no sign of any other weapon."

"And the murderer?"

"Is a tall man, left-handed, limps with the right leg, wears thick-soled shooting-boots and a grey cloak, smokes Indian cigars, uses a cigar-holder, and carries a blunt pen-knife in his pocket. There are several other indications, but these may be enough to aid us in our search."

Lestrade laughs and says, "I am afraid that I am still a sceptic." But Holmes is one step ahead of him. His friend, Dr. John Watson, is there to fulfill the role of reader, asking the questions we in the audience have but which are so basic that they would never occur to Sherlock to answer. Holmes explains how he deduced all the information about the murderer.

> "You know my method. It is founded upon the observation of trifles."
> "His height I know that you might roughly judge from the length of his stride. His boots, too, might be told from their traces."
> "Yes, they were peculiar boots."
> "But his lameness?"
> "The impression of his right foot was always less distinct than his left. He put less weight upon it. Why? Because he limped—he was lame."
> "But his left-handedness."
> "You were yourself struck by the nature of the injury as recorded by the surgeon at the inquest. The blow was struck from immediately behind, and yet was upon the left side. Now, how can that be unless it were by a left-handed man? He had stood behind that tree during the interview between the father and son. He had even smoked there. I found the ash of a cigar, which my special knowledge of tobacco ashes enables me to pronounce as an Indian cigar. I have, as you know, devoted some attention to this, and written a little monograph on the ashes of 140 different varieties of pipe, cigar, and cigarette tobacco. Having found the ash, I then looked round and discovered the stump among the moss where he had tossed it. It was an Indian cigar, of the variety which are rolled in Rotterdam."
> "And the cigar-holder?"
> "I could see that the end had not been in his mouth. Therefore, he used a holder. The tip had been cut off, not bitten off, but the cut was not a clean one, so I deduced a blunt pen-knife."

So much can be learned through thoughtful, proactive observation. We tend to forget that, especially today when we crave entertainment that allows us to think passively, to just watch, not to work too hard. It's not only Holmes' deductions that I admire but his confidence. He does not equivocate. This is a sign of years of study and application, consummate professionalism. This struck me as impressive when I read the stories as a child, and it is even more impressive to me now as an adult professional.

The deconstruction of Holmes' clues is a big part of the fun. In the end, I'm left with the obvious inevitability of his conclusions. The mysticism I felt at the beginning of the story is transferred from the deductions to the man making them. Holmes' powers of observation are extraordinary.

Yet for him, it's all in a day's work. His voice almost drips with boredom. Holmes understood that everything was important and so used all his senses. There was a reason those blades of grass bent like that. There was information in noting that the tip of the cigar had been cut, but not cleanly, rather than bitten off. Ash is not just ash, but a bi-product specific to a type of tobacco leaf from a certain place.

Everything is a clue. Details seem to wish to speak, yearning for us to understand them. The puzzle wants to be solved.

≥≤ ≥≤ ≥≤

I'm a physical therapist.

The term doesn't exactly ring with romance, and it certainly sounds less sexy than to call myself a detective. It's a medical field that doesn't get much attention. Fair enough that saving lives gets the headlines, but physical therapy (or physiotherapy elsewhere in the world) includes a wide spectrum of applications from brain injuries to wound care. My focus is on sports and orthopedics where I solve pain and help people return to their full potential. We may not be snatching patients back from the brink, but there is a lot to be said for fixing pain. There is a saying that goes "the healthy man has a thousand wishes, the sick man but one." The same could be said for anyone in pain. If you've felt physical discomfort for an extended amount of time, the one thing on your mind is how to stop it. There are types of pain that require medications and others that require surgical intervention. We help with those too, but my specialty is applying simple manipulations and shifts in habit, posture or movement which, almost magically, offer relief.

The mysteries I solve involve careful evaluation of patients. The moment I see them walk into my office I'm examining, evaluating, deducing. How they move, how they stand, how they sit can offer clues. Then there is what they say and any test results they bring, further shaking out puzzle pieces onto my desk, mysteries wishing to be solved. As we speak and as I examine them, I remain flexible in my deductions.

One of the "problems" with Sherlock's approach, as modern criminologists have pointed out, is that his deductions are always correct the first time around. If he sees a woman with a gold cross

Introduction

around her neck, he will deduce that she is religious. But what if her mother was religious and this was her necklace but the daughter is, in fact, agnostic? That doesn't happen to Holmes, but it happens all the time outside the borders of fiction. Holmes' murder suspect might have been left-handed, or might have been ambidextrous, or might have been carrying something in their right hand and so struck the victim with their left. Deductive reasoning requires flexibility and frequent resets and updates of hypotheses as new information comes forth. A patient might appear weak, and a doctor might suspect anemia, but a blood test shows that this is not the diagnosis, and so the hypotheses must shift. Holmes is a great inspiration but would not make for a good doctor.

A patient enters my office with baffling complaints of pain that have stumped other practitioners-as-investigators. They're looking for answers. If their pain is in the back or anywhere down to the foot, their walking pattern will be key to figuring out the mystery. The murderer in the Boscombe Valley Mystery might have limped because of a pain in his back, as much as being "lame," as Holmes concluded. If a patient's rib cage appears to slide down, or their knee points in or their hip juts out—it all has meaning. The body's ancient hieroglyphics are waiting to be read by someone who understands them.

If a patient's pain is above the waist, the clues I look for are found in how they use their shoulder blade, the shape of the thoracic spine, the rotation of the elbow. I find traces of rotations left at joints and study the lingering effects of their tension. The body and its movement (or lack thereof) paints a picture of behavior that has run amok and is now causing pain.

It all comes down to human behavior. That left-handed murderer had the habit of smoking his favorite brand of cigar, with a filter, and flicking his ash before discarding the butt. These are habits that are like tracks in the snow, leaving traceable trails if you know how to look.

With careful observation I can see these footprints, the ghost effects of the actual criminal I am hunting—the culprits behind pain.

After more than 25 years of practice as a physical therapist, the thrill of solving pain mysteries still excites me. I love seeing a patient who has baffled other practitioners. Our unique human construction demands that every case be considered differently. Even if I were to work with identical twins who lived together their entire lives, I would expect to see differences in their bodies. This is because the ultimate generator of pain and tension is the brain. Each person processes information differently, even if that information is identical. An early winter snowfall means different things to different people: one rejoices with thoughts of skiing, another weeps because they can't pay the heating bills, a third hopes school will be cancelled. Different reactions mean that tension patterns will differ too.

Like optical illusions in which some see a young woman and others an old hag, our brain "sees" in ways unique to an individual, like a fingerprint. Our brain senses and negotiates our environment through the five senses: smell, taste, touch, sight and hearing. These senses have a wide spectra of sensitivity and reach into our brain triggering domino effect repercussions in our minds and bodies. They result in behaviors. These behaviors are clues.

Although we are unique, pain is a shared experience. But rather than bringing us together in solidarity, we find ourselves separated in silent struggle to understand and rid it from our bodies. It is often lonely, especially without a cast or crutches to give us visible "permission" to hurt. It makes us feel that we are aging prematurely. It wakes us to our own mortality. In extreme cases, it can even make us wish to no longer live, if living means constant pain without promise of ebbing.

Pain is something we hide. We see it as a weakness, a failing of body, mind or spirit. In many cases, pain will resolve on its own. Sometimes it resolves because we've rested, bandaged, or avoided the activity that caused it. But in my more difficult cases, patients have robbed Peter to pay Paul. For instance, compensating for a flat foot by favoring the other foot leads to problems in the back. Subtle innocent compensations take their toll over time. Like taxes, inevitably they'll catch up to you.

None of these "criminals" show up on an MRI or x-ray. There are some suspects that would: a broken arm, a tumor. But when a doctor's arsenal of tests cannot locate the culprit, many medical practitioners are left scratching their heads in wonder and moving on to the next patient on their overloaded schedules. This is exactly the type of case a physical therapist is suited for—especially one who loves mysteries. And with about half of Americans seeking help for musculoskeletal pain, more than those who suffer from cardiovascular and chronic respiratory conditions combined, it looks like we're going to keep busy.

This book will help pull back the curtain to expose secrets of the body, debunk common medical myths and open your mind to new possibilities about pain and its relief. You'll learn to appreciate your body in a new way, pay attention to the clues it's trying to show you and become your own Sherlock Holmes.

⇛ 1 ⇚

The Reveal

The gentleman flew in all the way from New York to see me at my clinic in Colorado. It was the first time anyone had traveled extensively to see me, so I was taken aback. That's a long, expensive trip and I wanted to make sure I made it worth his time and effort. But the reason he'd come so far to see me was that his regular medical team was stumped.

In he walked or, rather, limped. He was in his late 60s, athletic of build. He loved to talk a mile a minute, and kept on smiling, punctuating his story with chuckles. He gave the impression that nothing could get him down. But here's the thing: he hadn't been able to straighten his knee for years. It all started after a minor surgery to fix a frayed piece of meniscus (a croissant-shaped piece of cartilage in the knee) that had been troubling him. But his problem was nothing you'd expect from a standard, simple surgery like that. He'd had x-rays, seen several doctors and physical therapists. There was nothing medically wrong with his knee, but no one had been able to help him.

There is a standard series of questions and basic but comprehensive examination techniques that I'll employ for every new patient, to get a sense of their baseline and to help identify what might be going wrong. A complete evaluation of the rib cage down to the foot is the starting point for any back or lower body problem at my clinic. Through the normal course of my exam, I would look at what I consider to be the usual suspects. I screen in a way that differs from most therapists, which can lead me to find things others don't. My basic screening distills the complex bio- and pathomechanics of the entire lower body system down to a few simple tests. A parallel is when a doctor orders a battery of blood tests, throwing out a large net to see if they can catch anything that shouldn't be there and could be a clue to the underlying problem. The clue then leads to further tests that home in on a diagnosis. I see my basic exam as a physical therapy version of this net. It's more comprehensive than most and I've found that it's been well worth it to spend extra time on the initial screening.

I spent years developing my screening net. As I put together complicated connections in the body, I would add a new strand. After a while, it looked more like a big tangle than a proper net, perhaps reminiscent of a child's drawing of a spider web, instead of the elegant construction you might see nature produce. But each strand was a possible way to catch a clue that would lead to a diagnosis and helping the patient. Like a spider, if something touched a strand, I knew immediately where the insect—in our case, the cause of discomfort—must be. As I approached the cause, I had this idea that it would struggle more, touching more strands as it did, and my certainty that I was correct in my diagnosis would strengthen. But then, unlike a spider that would trap its prey, I would do the opposite. Once I'd homed in on the problem, I would set it free.

Even though I knew he was coming to me after seeing a flurry of other professionals, I started with the basics so that I could get to know his body. Anything that would restrict knee straightening, like the hamstrings, are the first thought. The hamstrings (there are three of them: semitendinosus, semimembranosus, biceps femoris) cross the knee joint in the back of the knee on both the inside and outside, originating further up the leg or even the pelvis. Short hamstrings would then restrict the knee, keeping it from straightening, like a rope that isn't quite long enough. Surprisingly, his hamstrings didn't appear short at all. When I discovered this, a small ember of dread began to smolder in the pit of my stomach. This must have been exactly what the rest of his medical team experienced when examining him. Our default usual suspects all had alibis.

But shortness isn't the only reason the hamstrings might prevent your knee from straightening. They could also be in a protective spasm, guarding the knee for some reason that is not actually necessary. But his muscles were relaxed. No protective spasm and no shortness. Another dead end. I was doing what I imagined all those who had examined him had done, failing to find the reason, and the embers in my gut became a small fire. I inwardly scratched my head (perhaps outwardly, too, but even when you're stumped, showing your puzzlement doesn't inspire confidence in the patient).

Because the calf muscles also cross behind the knee joint in back, they would also be a potential candidate to restrict the knee. Yet his seemed to be relaxed and spasm-free when I tried to straighten the knee. Another potential suspect cleared of involvement.

Then I moved on to the internal structures of the knee that might restrict motion. The meniscus is the first that came to mind because small pieces can tear or be sheared off. These can block the knee from straightening or bending, like the small blocks you see holding a jet airliner's wheels in place when it's parked at a gate— it doesn't take much. Since the issue arose after meniscus surgery, this seemed like the next most likely culprit. The problem is that he'd had his meniscus repaired by a top surgeon in New York and he'd been assessed by other top doctors and PTs via a battery of standard orthopedic tests, endless MRIs and x-rays. Surely something would have shown up. But I found nothing wrong here, either.

Was the temperature in the room rising? I could feel myself starting to sweat.

I also tested his internal ligaments: the anterior and posterior cruciate ligaments (ACL and PCL respectively). All clear. Through all this, he kept commenting, "Oh yeah, I've had this test before," or he'd critique my technique: "The doctors cranked on my knee a lot harder than that!" He couldn't have been friendlier, but it only piled on the pressure, since I wasn't coming up with anything new. He'd been through all the obvious choices, had all the right tests. This was a puzzle of a case, for sure. I felt sympathy for his other practitioners—I knew exactly how they felt.

I maintained my calm outward demeanor but inside I was screaming at myself, "I can't let this man fly all this way for nothing!" I desperately wanted to reward his faith in me, the confidence he had that I really knew what I was doing. I needed that confidence in myself too.

It would be easy to write this off as "simple knee pain." After all, it's just a knee. How important could that really be?

That attitude unfortunately seems pervasive in medicine. "Oh, well, if I can't figure it out, at least it's not life threatening," and the practitioner moves on to a case they can solve.

Clearly, though, it was of the utmost importance to this gentleman—he'd spent years and thousands of dollars trying to solve his problem. It was a dark cloud hanging over his otherwise happy existence. I've learned not to minimize anyone's pain, nor its repercussions.

In medical mystery TV shows, like *House*, the doctors are stumped until our protagonist thinks laterally, outside the box. There are checklists we're trained to work our way through, and for almost every case we encounter, we'll hit upon the solution before we've exhausted the checklist. But that 1 percent of cases that stubbornly refuse to be solved even when we've run the gamut of usual suspect approaches and ailments are the ones that stand out, and that I find most interesting—the zebras. Sherlock Holmes didn't get excited by open-and-shut cases. If it looked like the butler did it, and the butler did indeed do it, then it didn't stretch his mental muscles. Here was a case that Sherlock would have gone for.

It would be fun if my life were like a TV show, like *House*, miraculously providing answers to difficult cases for me if I only observe "the signs." Unfortunately, that's not the case. It's sometimes messy and haphazard and agonizing. No, I have to figure it out for myself—as do we all.

So no muscles or internal structures seemed to be the culprit. What were all of us missing? Then it hit me in a flash. We had forgotten about one very tiny, and often forgotten, muscle.

⇒⇐ ⇒⇐ ⇒⇐

It had been a long day, a longer week and an even longer month. I was exhausted from an overloaded schedule. For the past two months I'd been on double duty, as one of my therapists left the clinic and I hadn't found a suitable replacement. My own patient load was such that I extended my hours to absorb her schedule. This was not early in my practice. I'd already been a physical therapist for more than 20 years. At this stage, I was hoping to slow down a little. Off and on I've struggled with depression throughout my life, and this was a period when it was creeping back up on me. Being overworked and overtired certainly didn't help. I was even questioning my decision to remain in this field. Sometimes things that you love and that you're good at can feel like a burden when life is getting the best of you.

Careers are supposed to have a constant upward trajectory. You start out modest and slope skyward, earning more money and accolades and solidifying your reputation until you plateau and then maybe take more time off and rest on your laurels.

Doesn't always work that way. Some careers just don't catch the public's attention, no matter how fascinating the people who practice them feel they are.

Although I owned a successful practice, the level of success, and especially my feeling of being successful, varied and swayed. I was in no danger of being invited on *Lifestyles of the Rich and Famous.* At the time, I drove a 20-year-old Subaru Forester that looked more like a golf ball on wheels than a car, its makeover courtesy of an apocalyptic hailstorm four years prior that gave its chassis a lunar look. I somehow had never gotten around to having it fixed or getting a new car. To be honest, at the time I couldn't afford it. My earnings went back into my clinic. I worked long hours, sometimes 12-hour shifts, to make sure everything ran smoothly. I was in danger of having a breakdown.

Anyone who runs a medical facility in the U.S. will know that helping patients is just one aspect of our workload. The most exhausting part is the labyrinth of frustrations and complexities that goes by the name of paperwork from insurance companies. There are many doctors who, when they reach a certain level, refuse to take patients who will pay through insurance because it's such a headache. The insurance companies try to pay out as little as possible, even when it's not in the best interest of the patient. A medical practice that relies on insurance payments can be like breathing through a straw—you just barely hang in there. It's a deal made with the devil: accept insurance contracts so you can see patients, but in doing so, you severely limit your income potential and play by the ever-shifting rules of insurance giants. Ask the insurance company to raise their reimbursement rate and they'll tell you to take a hike— there are plenty of other PTs itching for business.

So I breathed through that straw for years. I was burned out and starved for oxygen.

That's when Jeni appeared. She was a quiet, blonde-haired,

nine-year-old girl with oceanic blue eyes. In she limped, with her mother, Lisa, trailing behind. Jeni moved quickly, despite the limp, and it was clear she'd grown used to working around it. It was an odd injury. She couldn't straighten her left knee. It was frozen at a 30-degree bend. Imagine her leg straightening like clock hands: the upper part of her leg should point up at the 12 on a clock face, the lower part straight below it at the 6. In her case, her left leg was bent so that the lower part was stuck at 5 o'clock and couldn't make it to 6.

Jeni did her best to mask her limp. She walked on the tips of her left toes to make up for the length she'd lost due to her locked, bent knee. Her left hip was hiked high into the air to help unload the painful knee joint, which smarted when she put weight on that foot. She stared at me with a polite smile and steady blue eyes lacking confidence that I was her savior.

Jeni was an active girl who was involved in gymnastics, skiing, horseback riding and, at an informal level, wrestling with her twin brothers (she flexed her arm to show me her bulging biceps). She was precocious and had the firm handshake I might expect from a teenage athlete, not a nine-year-old.

Athletics had led to her current predicament. A month earlier she'd been running in gym class and had fallen, hitting her knee. The gym teacher reported hearing a loud, sickening "thump" when she hit the floor, and the whole room got quiet. An unnatural event in gym class. Not a good sign. Jeni was sprawled face down, unable to stand.

Her mother was called, and Jeni was taken to urgent care. X-rays confirmed that no bones were broken, but they found a bruise where the thigh bone met the lower leg bone.

At the knee, the long thigh bone splits into two lobes, called condyles. They are turned at slightly different angles. Through the magic of mechanical engineering, this allows for subtle rotation of the knee joint, as it bends and straightens. The inner condyle was bruised and would take time to heal. That wasn't her biggest problem at the moment.

The muscles around Jeni's knee had seized up and wouldn't allow her to straighten it. The hamstrings were most to blame. These muscles that run down the back of the thigh are very strong, designed for hard, constant work. When things go wrong, they can exert tremendous pressure on the knee joint. In Jeni's case, they locked her knee into that painful, bent position. She'd been stuck like this for just over a month with no change. Her method of accommodating had actually made it worse. Because she walked on the tips of her left toes, her left calf muscle, which crosses the knee joint, had also shortened.

I went through my examination, noting Jeni's elevated left hip and her inability to fully bear weight on her bent left leg. Throughout this process, I tried a few tricks, poking and prodding and gently massaging to find an open window that would lead to straightening her knee. All of my attempts were met with a silent grimace of pain. I was doing my best, my gentlest, but I was hurting this child patient of mine. She didn't make a sound or complain, but I could tell, and that, to me, felt like I was failing.

I was silently hoping that I wouldn't have to resort to forcing the knee straight. That would work, but it would be painful for her. And for me. I don't want to hurt anyone to help them.

Dramatically forcing a joint back into place is glamorized on TV but in reality it's a much different story. For example, with a dislocated hip, theoretically you should be able to pull the leg bone away from the hip socket to reset it back into place. Because of the size and strength of the muscles involved, a patient needs to be anesthetized to relax the muscles around the hip joint. Their spasm is actually preventing the hip from relocating, not to mention contributing to their pain. A knee would be a little easier as the muscles are smaller, but probably just as painful.

Jeni's case had echoes of a hip dislocation, due to the significance of the spasm involved in compressing the knee joint. The muscles just wouldn't let go until I said the magic word, whatever that magic word might be. But I didn't want to force the lower leg bone back into place. I would do all I could to avoid this traumatic last resort.

Jeni was my last patient at the end of that long day. The rest of the staff had gone home. Though it was mid–April, it was dark outside. Vivaldi's *Spring* played softly on the radio. It was the only positive vibe in the room. As my examination droned on, Jeni long lost interest in what I was doing. She rested patiently on her back and spaced out, staring into the patterns of plaster on my ceiling. Her mother Lisa's attention drifted away as she fiddled with her phone. I was on my own to figure this out.

I sat beside Jeni's left leg, keeping an eye on her face to see if anything I did caused discomfort. I needed to come up with something and I'd struck out so far.

Then I got an idea, more like a flash of inspiration. There's a muscle that is so small and unpopular and infrequently referenced that it's hard to believe it has any significance.

This is where my extensive training in anatomy from PT school must've kicked in. All those hours in the cadaver lab, month after month, teasing out the minutiae of muscles, nerves, ligaments and tendons. Where they run, their orientation relative to each other, how they interact with bones and so many other things that were lurking in the shadowy recesses of my memory, cobwebbed and waiting for me to find them again.

At that moment, I remembered having learned about this oft-overlooked muscle in school, but I couldn't recall the name. I did remember how it ran, its orientation and purpose. I held the lower leg bone, the tibia, just below the knee and gently pulled it towards me, away from her hip, to create a slight gap in the knee joint. I tried to exert only a pound or two of pressure, so as not to hurt her and trigger even more spasms in her muscles. I did this and included the slightest pressure to rotate the knee inward and offset the torque of this hidden, forgettable muscle the name of which, from that point on, I'd never forget.

The popliteus.

The popliteus is a thin strip of muscle that runs along the back of the knee from the inside lower leg bone, where it is thickest, to the outside thigh bone, where it is just a little tendon. It's small and deep and perfectly positioned to generate rotational torque in the knee joint. If I've learned anything in these past 20 years, it's that torque, or rotational force, often equals pain. While torque helps us translate power from one plane of movement to another, our bodies don't like to be stuck there. That's where Jeni's knee was, stuck in a torqued position that didn't show up on an x-ray.

Jeni's popliteus was locked in spasm and it had been for more than a month. This spasm, due to its rotational force, significantly increased compression at the knee joint which the muscles around were trying to guard against. It was like wringing out a rag: as you twist it, the distance between your two hands becomes smaller: compression.

The muscles around the knee didn't know they were contributing to the compression. They just knew that something was wrong and they were sentries on high alert. My rotation plus gentle massage released it, like letting go of one end of the rag. No more compression.

Jeni's thigh muscles and hamstrings began twitching softly like the fluttering wings of a moth trying to rise from the ground. And then they grew silent. Jeni's face gave no indication of pain as her knee slowly drifted down to the table, straightening. Was I imagining this? I maintained the pressure, cautiously tugging at her tibia while at the same time, unwinding the popliteus as her knee straightened further. Occasionally her thigh muscles quivered in weak protest and then silenced again. I almost heard them sigh as they gave up

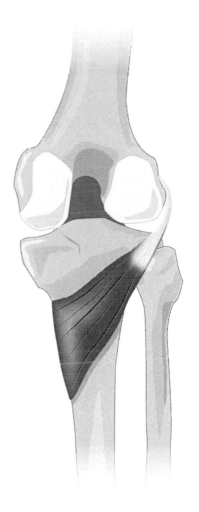

The popliteus, by virtue of its orientation, can twist the knee joint, creating pain.

their fight completely, once the back of her knee touched down. Their long battle to protect her was over—their silent retreat gave no indication of the violence of their origins. They'd gone home to rest.

Meanwhile, Jeni stared at the ceiling, bored and unaware of the quiet war we had just won.

Jeni's muscles had been caught in a reflex loop. Her knee was bent and slightly rotated, putting pressure on her bone bruise. This was painful and her muscles spasmed to protect the site of the pain. That was their job. But this caused more pressure on the bone bruise. Then her muscles responded with more contraction to protect the joint, which caused more bone bruise pain, which caused contraction to protect the joint and so on. I'd simply unloaded the site of the bone bruise to relieve the pain. This broke the reflex loop. The contraction was no longer necessary.

I looked up at her and whispered, "Hey, Jeni, check out your knee."

She lifted her head and did a double-take worthy of the Three Stooges. She stared in wide-eyed disbelief at her straight knee. I then saw a true smile on her entire face, not the half-smile indicating bravery in the face of adversity that she'd worn when she walked into my office. Her joy struck me like the soft brush of heat after you open an oven door on a cold February morning.

"Wow!" she whispered.

I turned to Jeni's mom. "Lisa, what do you think of this?"

Lisa had been immersed in her phone and only now looked up. Shocked by what she saw, she comically sputtered half-formed words, unable to utter a coherent sentence.

Finally, she said, "I can't believe it! What just happened? Is it really straight? Jeni! Can you see that? Oh my God, I'm about to cry!"

I almost teared up myself at their joy and relief. I felt like a magician who had just pulled off his big reveal to shock his audience. Voila! Except even I hadn't known how the trick would turn out.

Jeni got up from the table and, after a few tenuous steps, walked more confidently, with just a small limp that would go away in a day or two.

Lisa pulled me aside with moist eyes. "Jeni thought she'd never straighten her knee again. We weren't so sure ourselves. Thank you so much. What a session!"

My little magic trick for a nine-year-old girl and her mom proved to be just the thing. That moment, I was pulled back from a dark chasm. I felt my mind release. The reflex loop of my overwork and concern and depression let go. This didn't make everything right all of a sudden. I was still mentally limping. But it freed me from the trap I was in and set me on the road to recovery. All was right with the world, and I was lucky to be a physical therapist. Helping little Jeni led to her helping me rise out of my lowest moment.

≡≡ ≡≡ ≡≡

There he was, the gentleman from New York, lying on my table like Jeni had so many years before. I'd learned more than one lesson from her back then. Not the least of which was how, when the usual suspects are not guilty, you've got to think beyond the boundaries. Turn to the improbable, but not impossible. By now I'd found that the popliteus was behind some of the cases that stumped other therapists. It was rarely the only culprit, but instead slunk around in the background, letting the major players do their thing.

I ran my hand along the gentleman's leg, found the popliteus and massaged it for about five minutes. Physical therapy is not massage therapy, but massage is a key technique to uncoil taut muscles. Somewhere around the fifth minute I felt a palpable unlocking, like a thief feeling the tumblers of a safe. Boom, his knee straightened out.

I kept an almost bored expression that my hero, Sherlock, would've been proud of.

"Well, that seems about it," I said coolly.

He sat up, shocked to see his knee straight on the table. "What the ... how did ... huh?"

I'll be honest: sometimes my own tricks as a therapist-cum-magician delight and surprise me nearly as much as they do my patients. It keeps me on my toes never knowing when the "big reveal" is going to happen.

≋ 2 ≋

Summiting Migraines

Debbie, a longtime friend of ours, had been involved in a pair of automobile accidents that left her with chronic migraine headaches. She'd suffered for a few years before my wife convinced her that I might be able to help. It hadn't occurred to her that migraines could be caused by a musculoskeletal problem. But medication wasn't working well enough and wasn't a long-term solution.

If headaches are mountains, then migraines are like K2, the second highest mountain in the world. They aren't your run-of-the-mill headaches. They're fraught with all sorts of additional symptoms, including throbbing, nausea and even vomiting. They can include changes in eyesight such as seeing auras or blind spots. Similarly, tingling on one side of the face can linger for several days. Interestingly, they often occur on one side of the head. To me this is a key attribute.

In my simple way of looking at things, I see migraines as being on a headache spectrum—something that isn't mentioned in most research on headaches. Of course, at one end are the people who rarely get a headache, perhaps once a year, and it passes rapidly. On my headache mountain analogy, these people are out for a little hike in the foothills—some up and down but nothing too strenuous. And then somewhere in the middle there are those with diagnoses of tension headaches which are more frequent, intense and longer-lasting. These can range from the Appalachian Mountains to Mt. Kilimanjaro—the third largest mountain in the world. Getting closer to the other end of the spectrum are migraines and finally the ultimate is trigeminal neuralgia—the Mt. Everest of head pain and one of the most painful conditions in the musculoskeletal system known to exist.

Why do I see all of these on the same spectrum? Because my treatment approach to normal headaches also works very well for migraines. I've even helped the few cases of trigeminal neuralgia that have come my way. So the source of the problems seems to be very similar, if not the same. Instead, it's a matter of degree.

Migraines and trigeminal neuralgia both seem to happen mostly on one side of the head or face. Why would this be? In my experience, it's due to asymmetries in arm function due to handedness, past injuries that weren't adequately solved and posture patterns, such as having a rounded mid-back, faulty postural training and/or work-related postural issues. Of course, most medical practitioners will dismiss this interesting attribute as unimportant because they don't understand the connections between the arm and head or neck as a potential source of pain.

When I hear of musculoskeletal pain, no matter where it is in the body, as being unilateral, I automatically think I might be able to solve it. If it's on both sides this can indicate a more systemic origin such as a nervous system disorder, blood-borne disorder like a disease process, spinal disorder or some other issue not directly related to muscles, tendons and bone. That doesn't mean I won't try to help someone with bilateral symptoms; it just means my radar is turned to a high sensitivity in these cases to things that don't fit in to my treatment paradigm.

I was working out of our home at the time, so Debbie came by. After a few sessions her pain diminished significantly. She was pleased; I was pleased. This is where most physical therapists would stop. Quit while they're ahead, with a satisfied patient. Job well done, right? Well, sometimes I can't leave well enough alone.

I wanted to test to make sure she was truly better. So I got the bright idea to try to reproduce the stress of the accident. In our final session, I gently pressed on her left shoulder two or three times while she sat, mimicking the action of her seatbelt during those accidents. I used perhaps three to five pounds of pressure—not much. She didn't report any pain as I did this, so I figured all was well.

She called the next day to say her migraines had returned, and they were now worse than ever. I was dumbfounded. A delayed reaction, and now they were worse? I'm sure I spluttered something like "That's expected, don't worry." A classic stalling technique whereby

I hoped things just calmed down on their own somehow. Secretly I was completely stumped.

For three days I obsessed over her reaction. I could think of nothing else. Why had pressing her shoulder triggered her migraines? At the time I pressed her shoulder, I might've expected some shoulder pain or even some neck pain. But that it would trigger the worst migraine she'd had in years with such a gentle perturbation really threw me. Until that moment, I hadn't connected shoulders to headaches, only to perhaps neck pain at the most, which Deb had too. She could live with that, but the migraines were debilitating.

On the third day I had an epiphany. What if it wasn't her neck that was hurt after all? I still remember it clearly—it was almost like a religious experience. I was driving my car, vaguely paying attention to my surroundings, when a mental picture of the connections between the shoulder blade, neck and skull flashed into my mind. Once again, my extensive anatomical training in PT school came to the rescue. I instantly saw not only the physical connections but their implications for neck pain or headaches. I knew this was the answer—it explained it all perfectly to me. I couldn't wait to get home and look through my anatomy texts to confirm my vision! I was practically shaking with excitement and anticipation!

As far as car accidents are concerned, almost everyone has heard of the term "whiplash." Whiplash doesn't describe the tissues that are affected; it simply refers to the whipping motion of the head moving suddenly forward and back, as when a car abruptly comes to a halt, but your momentum continues to push you forward until the seatbelt stops you and throws you back into your seat. Rotation can be involved too, especially if the head was turned to see what that loud screeching noise was coming toward them. Considering that the human head weighs about 12–15 pounds, the physics of this type of accident becomes mind-blowing in terms of potential destructive power.

The problem is that the neck is a very complex and busy area of the body while also being vulnerable. The neck bones are the smallest in the spine because they need only support the head, instead of the entire upper body and trunk. The muscles and ligaments are smaller too and extensive, while balancing the head on top of the

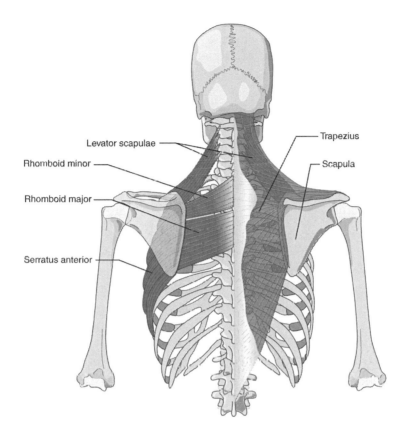

Levator scapulae

Rhomboid minor

Rhomboid major

Serratus anterior

Trapezius

Scapula

Connections between the shoulder blade, neck and head contribute to chronic headaches and neck pain.

neck. So a sudden jerk of the head can affect just about anything in this region.

Because there's so much happening in this area, up until that point, I hadn't considered that something other than the tissues found in the neck might have problems too. After all, everything below the neck is fairly stabilized with the seat and seatbelt.

Post-accident migraines can show themselves even many years after suffering whiplash. Treating her neck had soothed the migraines—my mistake was that I thought soothing meant solving. I had treated the neck and the symptoms went away, therefore the neck was the cause of her symptoms.

But the neck proved to be a red herring. By pressing on her

shoulder, replicating the force of the seatbelt upon her body during the accident, I unwittingly triggered the cascade of events at the root of her migraines—and they let us know loud and clear!

Current medical wisdom states that migraines are not completely understood but are caused by imbalances in chemicals in the brain, including serotonin, which regulates pain in the nervous system, and changes in the brainstem and how it interacts with the trigeminal nerve, which is the main highway for pain. The shoulder doesn't appear relevant to any one of the 10 most common migraine triggers named by the Mayo Clinic.

Fortunately, I didn't keep up with current medical wisdom as far as the causes of migraines. Not because I reject it, but because I'm engrossed in my little clinic identifying and following the strands of the web leading to pain. I generally don't accept "that's just the way it is." I've learned there's almost always a reason, even though nobody seems to have figured it out yet.

Going back to my anatomy books and studying the shoulder from a different point of view, I was able to see how the connections between the shoulder and the neck could lead to headaches and possibly migraines. The connections between our anatomy and their significance when it comes to pain and function were finally dawning on me. We learn this in a gross sense in school, which usually includes the actions of a muscle on a joint. But this new revelation went far beyond that for me, similar to the Butterfly Effect coined by the mathematician Edward Lorenz, which basically states that small changes in a system can have large ramifications further away from that source. These changes are often non-linear and therefore difficult to study or prove. But this understanding would forever change my approach to solving pain.

I thought I'd cracked the case.

I convinced Debbie to come in for one more treatment. Now that I looked at her differently, it was immediately evident that she couldn't hold her shoulder where it needed to be by herself. One of the things that tipped me off to this is that the dominant hand's shoulder should rest slightly lower than the non-dominant side. Debbie was right-handed but her left shoulder rested lower than her right. I hadn't thought this was significant because I didn't think the shoulder was significant. I was wrong. Reviewing the anatomical connections in my head, I visualized the stressors that must be acting on her skull.

Her doctors and I had been so focused on the neck that none of us had noticed her shoulder issue. I came up with a taping technique on the spot to hold it in place. She called the next day—no more headaches! Wow! It was as if I'd pulled off a magic trick, half-surprising myself. I thought it would work, but there's the lingering doubt until you try it, and then the delight in seeing that my theoretical mapping actually led to a real solution.

That was my first experience of the interplay between anatomy, movement and pain. The first of many. It strengthened my passion for finding the hidden pathways, ever expanding my knowledge so that I can reroute and solve pain.

≋ 3 ≋

Releasing Tigger

Years later, in my clinic, he was seated across from me, telling his story of eight years of sciatic pain. The man who sat in the wrong chair for 30 seconds and was in pain for a week after. His arms were folded across his chest, and his monotone voice ended with a drop in pitch, like Eeyore from *Winnie the Pooh*, saying, "If it is a good morning, which I doubt."

Al was a distinguished-looking 67-year-old in very good health, other than the feeling of numbness, offset by frequent stabbing pains, in his right leg. It was bad enough to send him to the emergency room on many occasions. His resigned, hopeless, Eeyore-like manner was the result of innumerable fruitless visits to a host of medical professionals. Cortisone shots to reduce a bulge they'd found in his spinal discs had failed to help him, as did surgery to remove some bone and part of a spinal disc. This offered relief for about six weeks. Then his pain returned, never to leave again.

Al struggled on. He had more tests to make sure the nerves exiting his spine weren't pinched. They were not. He was eventually told by a doctor that whatever it was would heal over the next two to three years. This is basically code for "We don't know what's going on. Let's wait and see if something shakes out." Another stalling technique from a stumped professional.

During those eight years, Al's lifestyle was negatively affected. He avoided things that triggered his pain, and that meant whittling down his life to keep pain at arm's length. The trade-off was that Al abandoned the small joys he once knew. This included spending time with his wife of 42 years, taking walks and shopping together. A simple trip to the grocery store was elevated to a serious review of the pros and cons of such an undertaking. He'd stopped working as a mechanical engineer. He couldn't lift, push or pull anything as a result of his sciatica. This included yard work, one of his favorite pastimes. Not only had he all but given up on medical professionals helping him, but he'd also given up on much that he enjoyed in life.

Al's pain pattern was typical of the sciatic nerve, a thick long cord that has its roots in the low back. Like an upside-down tree, the main trunk runs down the back of the leg, branching out along the way to supply the upper and lower leg muscles. This was the most obvious and most likely culprit for his suffering. When he walked, he felt pain and numbness in the toes of his right foot, the furthest branches of his sciatic nerve tree.

Lying on his back on my exam table, he lifted his leg while keeping it straight— Lasegue's Test. This looks for potential injury to the spinal roots of the sciatic nerve in his lower back. At my request, his eyes rolled, like my teenage daughter's do when my wife and I ask her to do something she'd really rather not.

"Okay," he sighed, knowing what we'd find. He raised his right leg a few inches off the table. "Oh my gosh, that hurts!" he said, through gritted teeth.

"Is that the pain you're complaining about?" I asked. "The pain you've been having all these years?"

"Oh yes, that's exactly what it is," he said, catching his breath after the lightning bolt that had just torn through his leg. His brow glistened with beads of sweat.

This confirmed that Al's nerve roots were pinched. No doubt other tests would also be positive for a source of problems in the spine.

But that was exactly the problem. Eight years' worth of various medical professionals had all come to the same conclusion. The simplest, most probable cause—the sciatic nerve. Therefore, to treat the sciatic nerve, you treat the lower back, and the problem would be solved. This was looking a lot like Debbie's problem. Her migraines and neck pain were assumed to be caused by a problem in her neck or head but were actually caused by her shoulder.

Likewise, it was assumed Al's pain was caused by his lower back. The question in my mind was "If not the lower back, where else?"

His treatment had focused on the spine the previous eight years. Certainly, if the problem was in the spine, the surgery, previous therapy, manipulations or cortisone shots should have cured it.

Solving the Pain Puzzle

I've learned over the years that, while many of these tests or treatments may reveal irritation at the spinal level, they do not pinpoint *why* that spinal level is irritated. This, it turns out, is the key to solving pain. Medicine is great at identifying structures that might be damaged or cause problems, but we tend to forget about asking why it is happening in the first place. So yes, it may be a sciatic nerve causing the pain, and the lower back may actually be bothering the sciatic nerve, but the question is why.

I finished my initial evaluation and found several problems, but I decided to cut to the chase. He'd been through a long line of health care professionals, each one certain they could help him. Al had heard it all before. I needed to do something dramatic that would demonstrate that his time with me would be well-spent. I needed another big reveal.

I asked Al to lie down on his back and raise his right leg again—Lasegue's Test, Round Two. With Eeyore's resignation, he raised it a few inches off the table. The result was the same searing pain tearing down his leg.

"Okay, remember how far up you can raise that leg and how much pain you're feeling," I said.

"Got it," he said, testing it one more time, his leg shaking. "It shoots right down my leg."

"Now roll over and get onto your elbows and knees," I said. He gave me a weird look—this, apparently, was not something any of the other eight years' worth of health care professionals had asked of him.

I had him lift his right leg up in the air with the knee bent and perform two sets of little pulses, to activate his butt muscles, the gluteals. He did this with some effort on his part. Then I asked him to lie on his back again.

"Now lift your right leg," I said.

He looked at me doubtfully, took a deep breath...

And his leg shot right up, almost perpendicular to the ground.

He was completely perplexed. I confess that I love seeing that look on people's faces. But even I was surprised at the extent and speed of the correction. My bored Sherlock Holmes expression remained planted on my face, however.

He lowered it again and repeated the leg raising about ten more times—no pain.

30

Al looked at me, no longer like Eeyore, but now incredulous. "Huh? What did you do?"

"I didn't do a thing," I said. "You did."

"I don't understand. How did that fix my back?"

"It's not your back that's the problem," I said. "It's your hip."

He pondered my words for a few moments. "But everyone's been telling me it's my back," he said. Then a longer pause before his inevitable next question: "Do you mean I didn't need to have that back surgery?"

"The back surgery may well have fixed problems in your back. But it seems those problems didn't relate to your pain," I replied. "It could be that the surgery removed a layer of problems that allowed this to work," I offered. The surgery may have been useless for the main issue. It may have been needed and useful for other reasons. It was difficult to say at that point.

"Then what's the problem?" he asked.

"You have a tracking problem in your hip joint that seems to be contributing to stress in your back."

Al had something called anterior femoral glide syndrome (AFGS), a fancy term meaning that the hip bone was moving around in the socket too much. When this happens, the bone usually moves forward, pinching tissue in the front of the hip. This is often diagnosed as a groin or inner thigh strain, or a labral tear. It can also cause hip bursitis, felt on the outside of the hip, due to the unruly thigh bone irritating a little lubricating sac called a bursa.

In the back of the hip, this often will be diagnosed as piriformis syndrome. The piriformis is a little muscle in the butt area that can irritate the sciatic nerve. Not surprisingly, this can irritate the entire hip joint, often attributed to arthritis. While these issues may be present, they are exacerbated by the poor movement of the thigh bone in the hip socket, causing them to feel painful.

AFGS is caused by poor butt muscle (gluteal) activity. The gluteals are primarily responsible for helping the thigh bone pivot correctly in the hip socket. When the butt muscles don't work well things get a little sloppy. I could tell just by watching Al walk to my table that his gluteals weren't working properly. This was confirmed during my exam.

Solving the Pain Puzzle

In Al's case I believe the head of the thigh bone migrated forward when he moved his leg, causing the piriformis muscle in the back of the hip to spasm. This then pinched his sciatic nerve as well as stressed the lower back due to a poorly controlled pelvic bone, resulting in his debilitating pain. Al's mechanical engineer mind grasped the information quickly.

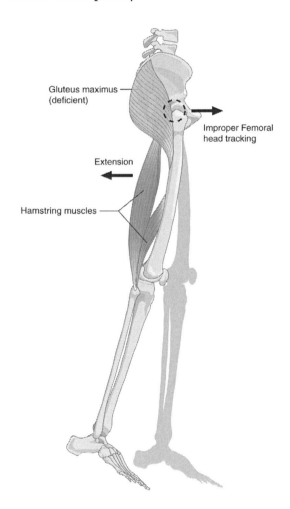

Anterior femoral glide syndrome occurs when the gluteal muscles do not function properly, causing the head of the thigh bone to migrate forward in the socket.

32

One of the things that tipped me off to his hip problem was something that Al *didn't* mention. Through all of my probing into his extensive history, Al never once mentioned he had back pain. Leg, yes. Back, never.

Al came back for his second visit a week later and was still pain free. But there was a second component to his issue that we hadn't addressed.

"But I still have this numbness in my lower leg when I use it a certain way, like moving something with my foot," he added. "What about that?"

"Show me," I said. I put an old phone book on the floor and Al slid the book with the side of his right foot. It produced numbness in his lower leg. He grimaced.

Al's sciatic pain was still gone. He'd been doing the exercises I assigned him to fix the weakness of his gluteals. Because his was a hip problem up to this point, I hypothesized that the origin of his lower body numbness wasn't coming from his back, either. So I performed a technique that used Al's own muscles to relax themselves around the right lower leg, foot and ankle.

The technique is called Hanna Somatics, a rather obscure approach that reduces muscle tension and reflexive spasming through controlled contraction and release. I spent three years studying this technique, which I like to say has become the jelly in my peanut butter and jelly treatment sandwich. The whole process took about five minutes. The result was like untying twine around a tightly wrapped Christmas tree and watching the branches fall loose again, assuming their natural shape. Al's muscles were able to move more freely, releasing compression of the branches of the sciatic nerve in his calf area.

"Test your numbness now," I said.

He moved the phone book— no numbness. I smiled at the look on his normally placid face. It was as if he'd just tasted chocolate for the first time.

He moved it more, scooting it across the floor. I held back a chuckle, watching this distinguished looking older gentleman express such delight at sliding a phone book around on the floor with his foot. Still no numbness. I added two more phone books on top of it. He moved those, too, without the feeling of numbness. He looked up at me.

"It's not my back," he whispered, half to himself. "After all these years, it's not my back."

As I watched Al's face, his eyes took on that unfocused look of someone who is thinking of something else while looking at me. I could almost see his brain synapses reconfiguring to align with this new reality. The image of a cocooned caterpillar that liquefies and reorganizes itself into a velvety butterfly came to mind.

To see those eight years of frustration and pain melt away from Al in that moment is one of the reasons why I love what I do. His face was a mixture of joy, relief and understanding. Imagine hurting for eight years. And then, suddenly, you don't. It can turn an Eeyore into a Tigger.

On Al's next visit I saw, in his relaxed confidence, the tone of his voice, his stride, that his new realization had settled in. Hope and understanding had been restored to his life. He was in control.

I then explained how Al got into trouble in the first place. This is important so patients don't slip back into bad habits. Remember, while Debbie had suffered a pair of car accidents, which were obvious precipitates for her migraines, Al had not been the subject of any particular trauma of which he was aware. I never learned of Al's precipitating event. For most it comes in the form of an auto accident, a fall, picking up a dirty sock, a yoga stretch, an extra mile of running that creates the dark solid pain.

His issue likely resulted from a slow burn of years of sitting at work in poor posture (and sitting too long), walking with poor technique and too little, performing the same exercise routine, sleeping in a slowly deteriorating bed, all of which enflamed very old injuries, causing joints to move a little less, muscles turning off just a little more. All of these tiny negatives accrue, like adding just a bit of a powder to a liquid until a solid pain precipitate emerges. So it is with how our bodies move. Problems crop up with a single severe incident (dumping a tablespoon of powder into a glass of liquid all at once) or very slowly (a few grains of powder at a time for decades). Either way, our movements have meaning and are often the keys to solving pain.

≡ 4 ≡

You'd Be Surprised

With something as finite as the human body, you'd think we'd know all there is to know about it by now. After all, our bag of skin has remained almost unchanged for tens of thousands of years. Yet our bodies are a never-ending source of investigation, wonder, pain, healing and exploration. Forget the infinite expanse of the cosmos or the unfathomable depths of the ocean. Just looking within ourselves will take us another thousands of years to unravel, so tightly are spooled our inner mysteries. We know so little about who we are. But we also know precious little of *how* we are.

My focus, as a physical therapist, is the musculoskeletal system. Most would think this the simplest system in the body to understand. It seems more finite than organs or neurons or cells, so we should have at least figured this part out by now, right? After all, we only have so many bones and so many muscles, don't we?

You'd be surprised.

Some people have an extra lumbar vertebra. Others are missing one. Some people have extra little rib nubs on their neck bones that most do not, called cervical ribs. Sometimes these are on one side, sometimes on both. Some have muscles that are absent in others. So, if you Google "how many bones are in the human body" and you receive the answer "206," or the number of skeletal muscles comes in at "650," just know that's not a definitive number.

Even if all the bones and muscles were known and constant, the variability in our bones' length and thickness means that some people have significant mechanical advantages (or disadvantages) due to the length of the lever arms their muscles act upon. And even if all of our bones were identical, where our muscles originate and insert into our bones has subtle differences rendering them stronger or weaker, depending on what you're testing. This is what allows one person to be a great swimmer while another is a great runner and a third is inept at sports altogether.

Of course, the master controller is the brain. If you think that there's variety in the body—in what should be our fundamental construction—then there are certainly infinite differences in our brains. These distinctions carry over to our control of our bones and muscles.

Consider a species of tree, say, an ash. Observe two different ash trees for even a few seconds and you'll see that no two are identical. Organisms are like snowflakes, each unique, even when they are the same species, even if they are twins. Within the same species of any living thing, you'll find variability. In humans, that variability creates differences in wear and tear on bones, muscles, ligaments and tendons.

At first glance, the musculoskeletal system appears as if we're all basically built the same. Well, that's what I thought upon entering physical therapy school in 1994. I assumed that everything had been worked out by researchers past, that there were no new mysteries to solve, at least about injuries and pain. After all, how hard can it be to understand how we move?

Turns out that the question may not have been how hard it is but instead where to focus our attention. As a profession, physical therapy over the years became more interested in defining the smaller parts of our body, like the forces delivered to the meniscus (a piece of cartilage in our knee) while pivoting, than how exactly we go about pivoting. Or the amount of compression felt by the discs between our vertebrae when bending forward, rather than *how* we're bending forward. To me, the "hows" of human movement feel more pertinent than knowing the exact newtons of force these tissues are experiencing or whether a millimeter of movement has occurred at a joint.

I'm an orthopedic physical therapist, and my job is to solve pain and improve function. Early on in school, it seemed to me that understanding how we move is central to this job. I learned, during school and most of my career, that this part has been largely skipped over. At the time I thought I'd simply missed this key information— that I had somehow fallen asleep during that class. This created significant anxiety in me as I prepared to graduate and land my first job as a PT. It didn't help that my classmates, all much smarter than me, appeared unconcerned to be released into the wild.

After some struggle, soul-searching and a significant battle with depression early in my career, I set off on a quest to learn how it is we fit together to create and solve pain. After reading some of the stories in my book, many of you might think, "But he hasn't included Treatment X"—you can pick any type of treatment that I do not touch upon. There are, indeed, infinite variations that can occur in our bodies, and there are myriad depths of problems at the roots of human pain. Not all cuts need stitches, even though stitches help cuts heal. Some people's problems might be shallow dips in a path, while others are deep holes they can barely see out of. This book is my way of showing how I helped people out of the deeper pits that they couldn't climb out of themselves, no matter how many medical professionals threw them lines to pull them up. Their issues required a deeper understanding of how and why we have pain. You don't call in Sherlock Holmes for an open-and-shut case. You call him in when you're stuck, when hope is at its dimmest. This isn't an encyclopedia of methods; it's a selection of stories of medical mysteries and how, with the right information, they unraveled. Most of the stories are now complete. With an understanding of their habits' role in their pain, these patients now think of the solutions as surprisingly simple, practically effortless. The common refrain from my patients is often "I don't feel like we really *did* much, but now I'm pain free." That's music to my ears. Education about why there is pain is integral to my program. Knowledge is power. It means that my patients almost never slip back into bad habits.

Some of you reading this enjoy medical mysteries. Others are aspiring health or wellness professionals interested in exploring some of the tougher cases of our field. But I'd guess that most of you reading this are doing so because you are a patient with some chronic or nagging pain that just won't to go away. You've tried your family doctor, maybe even a specialist or two, without luck so far. My greatest hope is that you think of the following stories of pain, diagnosis, therapy and relief as clues to solve your own pain. But they are not only clues. They are a whole new way of thinking about how your body operates. I hope to inspire you to take a lesser-known path and rekindle that inner fire to find your solution. The solution is there. It's just a matter of shifting your thinking, putting on your Sherlock Holmes hat, and looking where others have not. I'll be with you every step of the way.

I'll Have Mine
with a Twist

"Ride with your knees a quarter to a half inch further from the frame," I said, "and rotate your shoe cleats out about two or three degrees. Lastly, start walking with your feet turned out a bit."

"You mean walk like a duck?" Brian, my new patient, asked incredulously.

"Yes, if that's how you want to think about it," I answered.

"When can I ride?" asked Brian, a lean 31-year-old with the shredded thighs of an elite cyclist. He'd raced in many countries around the world and he was now training for the Colorado Classic, a multi-stage, multi-day road race ranging from about 90 to 130 miles of riding each day through the steep, winding valleys and passes of the Rocky Mountains. This was one notch that this Colorado native hadn't yet put in his belt, and he felt it was time.

Brian had been training for months for this race, but his efforts had ground to a halt due to stabbing right knee pain that developed three weeks earlier. He consulted Dr. Google (as the search engine is affectionately called by medical professionals) and had tried what the good doctor had suggested: rest, ice, stretches and various salves, ointments and over-the-counter medications. All to no avail.

All my patient examinations begin with them standing and facing me while I take in the big picture of the body they've brought in that day. Brian stood there in his shorts, with veined, shaved legs and bulging muscles around his knees. His feet pointed straight ahead, and he had high arches. This is referred to as foot supination, as opposed to foot pronation, which is low or flat arches. Like I do with all my patients, I examined him from rib cage to foot to understand his particular architecture as well as the stressors working on it.

Brian was an athletic specimen and, not surprisingly, had no discernible weaknesses or abnormally tight muscles. Everything tested out perfectly, as I suspected it would.

However, there was one twist (literally) in his structure that could explain his pain. Brian had retroverted femurs—thigh bones that were twisted outward a little more than normal. Like most things in the human body, there is a spectrum along which each person falls. In regard to thigh bone shape, some are twisted outward, like Brian's retroverted femurs, and some are twisted inward, called anteverted femurs, like those of Satori, a patient you'll meet later. This is a naturally occurring phenomenon. I've found that men typically develop retroverted thigh bones, while women typically develop anteverted thigh bones.

A common observation/complaint that I hear is that men typically sit with their knees apart. Often this is judged as unappealing. Women, on the other hand, sit with knees together—a more culturally acceptable manner. But I've come to believe that men and women have a general tendency to sit in these differing ways due to the shape of their thigh bones—it's natural for men's legs to spread apart because of this retroverted twist. Likewise, it's more natural for women to sit with their knees together, an act made easier by the anteverted twist in their thigh bones.

Of course, some women have retroverted femurs and some men have anteverted femurs. Some have one retroverted femur and one anteverted femur. This was the case of an NFL lineman, Carl, who came to me with chronic right-side hip pain that began during his college days and would manifest during his pass sets, when he would back up to create a protective pocket for the quarterback. He was a right tackle and was taught to slightly internally rotate his right leg (pointing his knee gently inward) while planting his right foot behind him, to create an unmovable post. The problem was that his right thigh bone was retroverted, rotated outward. This meant that he had less available inward rotation in that hip or knee joint, so asking him to slightly internally rotate his leg forced him to use up all his available internal rotation, which was very little anyway.

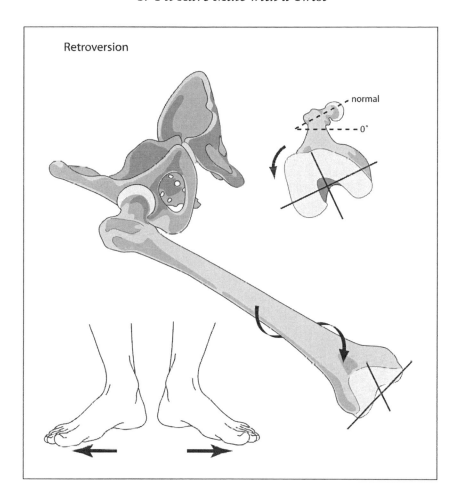

Retroversion

normal

0°

Femoral retroversion, where the thigh bone twists outwardly, occurs naturally. This is more common in males.

Internal rotation in any joint in the body, especially at the hip,
knee and shoulder, increases joint compression, and therefore tissue breakdown and pain. Carl tested positive for a labral tear in his
right hip joint—no surprise there given his profession and its necessary mechanics. But that wasn't the cause of his pain. It was the fact
that his coaches had trained him to internally rotate his right thigh,
unaware that this recommendation was actually weakening his ability to post that leg, rather than strengthening it. This, combined with

the forces he was absorbing to protect his quarterback, was his recipe for pain.

Carl had three options. First, he could allow the right leg to remain slightly rotated to the outside, in order to maintain proper alignment based on the shape of his thigh bone. Second, he could strengthen his gluteal (butt) muscles. The gluteal muscles help externally rotate the thigh bone and therefore would reinforce his coach's instructions by countering or decelerating internal rotation of the thigh bone he was supposed to use in that situation. Or third, he could move positions, switching to the left side of the line, favoring his left femur, which wasn't retroverted, and consequently handle internal rotation better.

Due to his unique job, and the fact that he couldn't change sides of the line just based on the shape of his thigh bone, we decided to adopt solutions one and two. I gave him a gluteal strengthening exercise and tasked him with practicing his pass sets with less internal rotation of his thigh bone. On our next visit, a few days later, he complained of how sore his butt muscles were. He had never isolated them before. His training mostly included multi-joint strengthening exercises to prepare for the rigors of his job—not isolating specific muscles. He also reported his right hip pain was reduced by 75 percent.

Turns out that the remaining 25 percent was due to his tight soleus muscles controlling his foot and ankle. The soleus muscles lie deep to the calf muscles and originate about halfway up the lower leg bone in the back. Along with the calf muscles, they blend into the Achilles tendon to insert into the heel bone. The soleus muscles need length to allow the ankle to bend. Carl's were too tight, and therefore his ankle couldn't bend properly. In these situations, the forces trying to bend the ankle have two options: they can cause the foot to flatten excessively, contributing to a variety of foot ailments, or they can transfer the forces back up to the knee, which then has to deal with the problem. Carl's body chose to throw the problem back up to the knee, which was trained to follow the internal rotation of the thigh bone which, in turn, passed the forces into his right hip—another contributor to his right hip pain.

To tackle this (sorry, couldn't resist the pun), I gave him a soleus stretching exercise and we incorporated soleus lengthening into his training regimen to reinforce the new length we were asking of the soleus and foot and ankle. On his third visit, he reported that his hip pain was basically gone. A good thing, given that training camp started in two days.

⇒⊏ ⇒⊏ ⇒⊏

"You can ride today if you want," I replied to Brian. "Let's see how it goes."

Brian left my clinic with a puzzled look on his face, after my recommendation to turn his cleats out a couple degrees and let his knees rest away from his bike frame another quarter to a half inch. He was especially confused when I said that, to top it off, he should walk with his feet turned out a little.

I'm used to those looks.

A big part of cycling is drafting, when the cyclist tries to remain in a streamlined position behind other riders, to avoid head winds. This involves tucking as much of the body into one's center as possible—internal rotation of most joints—a recipe for injury for those whose bones are not designed for internal rotation, like Brian's.

Allowing his knees to drift outward a little may not exactly change the amount of internal rotation of his thigh bones much, but it will certainly change the force he's using to keep them close to the bike frame. Sometimes a little decrease in force is all that's needed, especially when you're talking about tens of thousands of repetitions, as is the case with cycling. Turning the bike cleats out a few degrees would introduce a second layer of force reduction, stripping torque from the knees and hips by aligning the feet with the shape of his thigh bones.

Recall that Brian pointed his feet straight ahead when he stood and walked, but his thigh bones were rotated outward. People with retroverted femurs need to turn their feet out to match the rotation in their thigh bones. If they don't, torque is introduced into the system because one part of the leg, the thigh bone, is trying to rotate outward while another part, in this case Brian's feet, were rotating inward, relative to his thighs. In essence, he was trying to override the shape of his thighs to accommodate a socially acceptable ideal that all feet should point straight ahead.

They shouldn't.

Torque, in Brian's case, played out in his knee. It could've just as easily manifested as pain in his feet, ankles, hips, sacroiliac joint (the junction in the pelvis where the broad ilium meets the sacrum), pelvis or lower back.

Feet with high arches are uncommon. Brian's high arches, together with the fact that his feet were pointed forward, alerted me to the possibility that he was artificially adopting his current stance. This was confirmed when he commented that he would be "walking like a duck" by turning his feet out. This is a negative judgement about how he should be standing or walking, rather than an acceptance of how his body is built.

Brian came into the clinic a week later looking a little down. Prior to this, he complained that could ride only two miles before his stabbing knee pain began. I didn't have a good feeling. Had my approach failed?

"I did what you said and went out for a ride the afternoon after my last visit. At two miles, I had no pain, so I decided to try five miles. Still no pain, so I did ten miles—no pain. I ended up riding forty miles on hills and had no pain!" he said, smiling.

"Why the long face when you came in, then?" I asked.

"Oh, I was just messing with you!" he laughed. "I can't believe it! So simple! You solved it!"

⇒⊂ ⇒⊂ ⇒⊂

Understanding thigh bone rotation and its implications is critical to solving most lower body and back pain. At the other end of the spectrum, internally rotated thigh bones (femoral anteversion) cause problems too.

This was the case of Satori, a woman who flew in from Washington to see me. She explained that she had been born with a severe right hip deformity which caused her right leg to be three centimeters shorter than her left. She didn't want to stand out, so she'd tried her best not to limp ever since she was a young girl. As a result, she'd worn out her left hip and had a hip replacement 11 years earlier. Then, seven years later, her deformed right hip was replaced, a procedure complicated by a history of reconstructive surgeries for that hip. She reported that she'd had "crazy" left hip pain these last few months. She'd been through the usual host of tests and practitioners

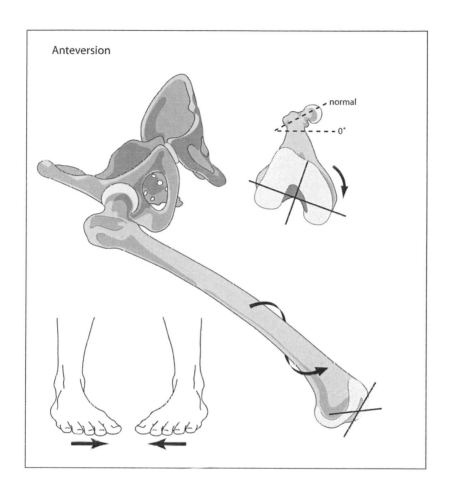

Anteversion

normal

0°

Femoral anteversion, where the thigh bone is twisted inwardly, is the opposite of femoral retroversion and is found more commonly in females.

and was desperate to stop her pain, which kept her up at night and lasted throughout the day. Her pain was in the front, back and side of her left hip.

I evaluated her as I did Brian and found that her knees rotated inward excessively, and she had flat feet. She walked by locking her knees straight. I discovered that she had an elevated left side of her pelvis and her left rib cage rested lower than the right side (I describe this as a "depressed rib cage").

Her walking pattern was unusual too. Her right rib cage shifted down when she stepped on her right foot and, at the same time, she hiked her left hip high into the air to swing her left leg forward. Based on her history, this could have been a very old pattern she adopted when she was young, to compensate for her right hip deformity. She had poor gluteal muscle activity and weakness. I also found she had internally rotated thigh bones (anteverted femurs). Lastly, I found that she had a problem with her new hip joints, which moved in their sockets incorrectly—Al's problem in Chapter 3.

After examining her, I was sure I could help.

Since she'd flown in from out of state, she blocked off the entire week to see me and we had three sessions to fix everything. I like to put at least a day in between sessions to give people a chance to try out my recommendations and see how they respond.

Our first job was to level her pelvis and rib cage. I use a powerful technique learned in my Hanna Somatics training to do this. It takes about 10–15 minutes and then I gave Satori exercises to maintain the level pelvis and rib cage. This is a key test for my patients. It's very easy to keep a pelvis and rib cage level once they've been corrected. If, when I see them next, they're not level, I know they haven't been trying hard to help themselves, at which time I become very stern. I prefer to work with people who will try to help themselves.

I also taped the backs of her knees to stop her from locking them. This is critical to establishing a therapeutic gait pattern. Locking the knees disrupts normal muscular activation throughout the lower body and back and is a habit that must be stopped.

Satori didn't disappoint me. Her second session began with my confirmation that her pelvis and rib cage were level. She reported that she felt about 65 percent better and had slept through the night with no pain. Great! When I see a large jump in pain reduction, it confirms that we're on the right track.

Next, I dealt with her butt muscle strength and timing by giving her a targeted butt strengthening exercise like Al's. I taught her to improve her walking pattern to turn on her all-important gluteal muscles too. This was critical because these muscles would prevent her thigh bones from rotating inward, help maintain a level pelvis, and improve how her hip bones were moving in her hip sockets. If

46

the thigh bones can be controlled, then the knees won't collapse in excessively and this will unload foot flattening forces.

She was motivated, especially feeling so much better already. Her quick smile and laughter made working with her a pleasure—we were having fun.

Feeling hopeful, she then brought up that her left arm had been numb for several weeks and she wanted to fix that too. She hadn't mentioned it before, as she didn't think we'd make so much progress in a day. I took a quick look at her arm and taped her shoulder blade similar to how I taped Debbie's in Chapter 2. It is common for patients to start asking me about a bevy of other aches and pains once their main problem resolves. I don't mind at all: it's a sign that things are working better and that they trust me.

On our third day, she reported only a slight ache in her left hip—virtually no pain at all. Her left arm had just a small bit of tingling in it too. We fine-tuned her walking pattern to make it even better. I checked her hip joint motion and found that it had improved significantly. Finally, I confirmed that her pelvis and rib cage were still level. I then gave her an exercise to improve her shoulder blade strength, now that I knew that this was the source of her arm numbness.

She flew home later that day, but she still drops me an occasional email, thanking me and letting me know that she's still pain-free, now more than five years after her week-long visit, as long as she continues walking to control her rotating thigh bones and unruly hip joints. Her story is a valuable reminder that complicated problems don't necessarily need complicated solutions.

This underscores the reason that I'm sharing these stories. Chronic pain is rampant in the United States and around the world, resulting in an opioid crisis, lost wages, decreased productivity and, perhaps most importantly, lost family time. What if we could solve these problems before they ever became serious? What if coaches, gym teachers and trainers understood things like retroverted or anteverted femurs? Or dancers and gymnasts understood how depressed shoulder blades lead to chronic neck pain or headaches? Or doctors and physical therapists learned to understand how the legs are the primary stressors creating back, SI joint or sciatic pain?

The stories in this book often depict "miraculous" recoveries. That is not the exception at my practice; it is the rule there. We're in the business of miracle recoveries, but it's not due to miracles. It's about a deep, considered knowledge of the musculoskeletal system. Each body is a puzzle that I love to solve.

Knowing how quickly the body responds to the right things helps me move rapidly as a therapist solving pain mysteries. If I don't see at least a 30 percent or more decrease in pain after our first visit, I begin to think I might not be on the right track. If, by the second visit, someone's not 50 percent better, assuming there are no other extraneous medical complications, then I begin looking somewhere else for the potential source of pain. In my practice, I expect to solve body puzzles and ease pain in a way that patients consider miraculous, based on their previous experiences.

That's the beauty of understanding the human body from a systems standpoint, one that sees problems simultaneously from micro and macro levels: rapid identification of problems and rapid results. My method hinges on two core beliefs: First, pain is an indication that something is wrong right now, and second, our bodies have many self-repair mechanisms in place to assist us in healing. This is the only way I can explain why so many people feel better so rapidly once those obstacles are removed.

Hopefully, you're getting the picture that there may be answers for your pain too.

≋ 6 ≋

Ground Wires

When I was about 11 years old, growing up on our farm in Ohio, we had a cheap little toaster oven that sat on the kitchen counter next to the fridge. Every now and then we'd get to have an English muffin as a change from our usual Wonder Bread. I used to look through that half-burned glass to watch it toast, waiting to slather on the butter.

One day I came home from school and saw it sitting in the trash bin out in the garage.

"Why's the toaster in the trash?" I asked Mom.

"It's broken," she said.

Though I loved toast, this was the best news I'd heard in a long time.

I immediately snatched it from the bin and scuttled back to my bedroom. There I had an old red desk that served as my tinkering bench. It was like Christmas morning! Secretly I loved taking apart my toys to see how they worked. This was my first chance at a real adult appliance. I grabbed some of Dad's tools from the basement and set to work.

I removed the back panel and saw where the electric cord entered the toaster. After careful study, I noticed one wire suspended in the air. On the back panel, there was a weld spot with a little nub sticking out of it, just like the wire that was waving around. I lined them up and, sure enough, it was a perfect match. It was the ground wire.

My big sister had a phase then of making stained-glass ornaments. She'd set up a little studio for herself downstairs in the basement. I used to watch as her soldering iron magically melted metal, only for that metal to solidify again once the iron was withdrawn.

49

Solving the Pain Puzzle

I was under strict orders not to touch it—ever.

In spite of this commandment, that afternoon her soldering iron dripped large gobs of solder on that broken metal tip inside our toaster oven, securing it back to the frame. That sucker was never going to come free again.

I then plugged in the toaster oven, flipped on the switch and saw the heating coils turn red—it worked!

I quickly put the panel back on and brought the refurbished toaster oven out to the kitchen counter. I stuck two pieces of bread in and turned it on.

Mom was sitting at the table reading a magazine.

"Hey, Mom, want some toast?" I blurted out.

For many months thereafter, every time I—or anyone else, for that matter—used the toaster oven, I would swell with pride.

That toaster was the beginning of my understanding that there's a logic to how things work. I saw that, while these connections were often hidden from view, with a little curiosity and work, I could figure them out and fix them if they were broken.

After I graduated from the Ohio State University with a degree in science education, I applied my fondness for tinkering to a broken-down motorcycle that I used to explore Australia in my early 20s. I couldn't afford a mechanic, so I would often camp by the side of the road in the Outback and practice taking apart the carburetor, memorizing where each screw went. At the time, I was reading *Zen and the Art of Motorcycle Maintenance* by Robert Prisig, which actually gave me a few clues as to how think about all this.

It was a time before mobile phones or the Internet, so it took me a while to understand things. I largely had to figure them out on my own—no instructional YouTube videos. Eventually, because my bike was so run-down, I relented and brought it into a bike shop. I explained that I was traveling around Australia and needed to learn how to fix this thing and that I wanted to watch what they did. I could only afford one visit to memorize everything. They were happy to oblige.

I discovered the role of floats in a carburetor and how to adjust them to keep the gas/oxygen mixture just right, to clean the gaskets that were prone to collect fine dust from the road and to remove and check the tubes feeding the carburetor. It was all very logical and satisfying to me on a deep level. That visit exposed the mystery of the engine and, from then on, I felt comfortable exploring further, knowing that I could put back together whatever I dismantled.

I managed to make it to Western Australia over the next several months tinkering with my bike along the way to keep it going. I needed to fix a new problem there, but I didn't have the right tools. So I found another motorcycle repair shop, this one in Perth, and I asked to use theirs. I removed my gas tank and carburetor within minutes while the owner watched.

"Hey mate," the owner said, "how long you been fixin' bikes?"

"Oh, about two months now," I said.

His eyebrows went up. "You serious?" he asked. His other two employees were listening now.

"Yeah," I said. "Had to figure it out cause this bike is such crap."

"Wait, you're not a mechanic?" he said.

"No, I'm just tooling around Australia," I replied.

After another minute of watching me, he said, "Mate, you want a job?"

I didn't imagine my future as a motorcycle mechanic in Perth, Australia (though, come to think of it, that sounds pretty sweet). But I was flattered and inspired by my ability to understand the inner workings of things, to recognize what wasn't functioning as it should, and to make it better.

I came home from traveling those many years and moved to Boulder, Colorado, where I worked various jobs. After some months there, a friend mentioned that her dad was in physical therapy for an ankle problem. I had never heard of physical therapy. I learned that it's a combination of medicine and exercise. I liked both of those fields and decided to check it out.

I volunteered at a sports and orthopedic clinic to learn more and fell in love. I saw therapists doing interesting things with people, handling different parts of the body in mysterious ways. People left feeling better. The therapists gave them exercises, critiquing or modifying them. I suppose on some level this spoke to my mechanical affinity for figuring out how things worked and fixing them.

My undergraduate grades at OSU weren't good enough to apply to PT graduate school. I had to take a few prerequisite courses to round out my application. But with my new enthusiasm, I received all As in my pre-req courses. Even so, I was happily surprised that University of Indianapolis let me in given the fact that the bulk of my science coursework was almost 10 years old and that my time off from school meant I was now a non-traditional older student. I was a risk.

While I wasn't the best student by a long shot at U of I, I enjoyed most of the classes. I learned so much and it all fascinated me. I often had to pinch myself to be sure I wasn't dreaming! I loved my anatomy classes best of all. To see our inner workings fascinated me. My classes in sports and orthopedic rehabilitation, while interesting, left me unsatisfied. I learned about strains, tears, broken bones, how they heal and what to do, but I had a nagging feeling that something was missing. I couldn't place my finger on it. I grew anxious as school continued.

There seemed to be a piece (or many pieces) missing for me. It was as if I were being taught the beginning of the equation—the anatomy, physiology, etc.—and then there was the end of the equation—progressing people through exercises—but there was a big chunk in the middle that seemed to be missing. Yet my classmates apparently understood this middle chunk or didn't notice the gap. How did that anatomy and physiology translate into pain or fixing that pain? Had I missed a key course in school?

Upon reflection, I think that I was missing the "why" behind it all. Today, this is the key to my approach. I search out and fix the why's—I find the butterfly whose wings are flapping causing a hurricane across the globe. Once the butterfly's wings are tamed, the hurricane hushes.

〓〓〓

At graduation, one of my classmates came up to me and said, "Rick, I've never known whether you're the smartest guy in the class or the dumbest." I hadn't realized that it was so obvious to others.

I certainly never felt like the smartest which is why I often didn't express my concerns to my classmates—I didn't want to highlight the fact that I felt out of my depth. In fact, I was somewhere at the back of the peloton and, as graduation loomed, I was in a near panic. There was still so much I needed to learn! I felt unprepared to be a proper PT but I didn't know why. I simply had a general feeling that something was missing. It was like a secret had been passed to them that I'd somehow missed. What did they "get" that I hadn't?

I landed my first job as a sports and orthopedic physical therapist in the small town of Cortez, tucked into the southwest corner of Colorado. Luck seemed to dictate my patients' outcomes more than anything. I was basically on my own, with no mentor to show me how to help them. It showed. Every day I dreaded facing my patients, knowing that I didn't have the answers they were seeking. The fear I felt upon graduating bore out in the clinic. To put it simply, I felt I should be doing a better job.

It didn't help that I replaced a PT, Bret, who apparently worked miracles and whom everyone loved. I could never live up to his reputation.

In terms of my early failures in Cortez, there was a particular patient, Robyn, who stands out in my mind. Bright and full of smiles, young and athletic, she'd had ACL repair surgery. Things were going great until at about eight weeks, when she developed knee pain in her surgical knee. I assumed it was my fault: after all, I was her PT. No matter what I did, I could not get that pain to go away—I tried everything I knew. I asked other PTs and tried what they said. Her doctor confirmed that nothing was wrong with his surgery. She came back again and again for help but nothing worked. She haunted me.

Another patient with back pain was a young mother of two and very athletic. She could do back bends where her hands and feet were both on the floor. But nothing I tried helped. I drove six hours to Denver to take a back pain course one weekend, mostly with helping her in mind. I came back only to find none of the information I'd learned worked with her. Again, she looked to me for help, but I had none to give, despite my efforts.

These people and others looked to me for answers I didn't have. I thought of them daily, seeing their expectant faces searching mine for an answer. I could only stare back blankly—no answer, no wisdom, no understanding to offer them.

After that first year, I considered quitting physical therapy— clearly, I just didn't have what it took. But I had only recently graduated and spent so much time, effort and money on my education that I couldn't give up, at least not yet. I'd become a physical therapist to help people. It's what I felt I should be doing. I loved learning about how we worked. So I did what I did best at that time of my life and decided to travel, to think it all through. I bought a round-trip ticket down to Costa Rica for three weeks, which was fabulous.

I trekked through the mountains and volunteered for a leatherback turtle project in a small village without electricity on the country's east coast. Leatherbacks are huge, like oversized ottomans waddling around. My work involved patrolling the beaches during the night to ward off turtle egg poachers. While I explored Costa Rica, Spanish from a lifetime ago in college came back to me.

In spite of the beautiful beaches and gigantic turtles, there was a dark cloud hovering over me. "What will I do when I return? I'm not a good physical therapist." The very thought of working with patients again filled me with dread and anxiety.

My three weeks were up, and I was no closer to knowing what my next step would be. So I threw away my return ticket. Instead, I traveled overland through Central America and Mexico for the next six months. I didn't realize I was developing a mild form of PTSD. I would replay my failures in my head again and again with nothing else to think about. This sank me into a greater depression.

But there were many distractions from my quandary. The people of Central America were warm, friendly and tolerant of my Spanish. The markets were colorful with delicious foods, like plantains and a world of spices that reminded me of my world-wanderings when I was younger. My visits to ancient Mayan ruins like Chichen Itza helped put my problems into perspective. Right or wrong, a bigger picture started emerging of these once-thriving cultures being driven apart or simply melting away, absorbed by some other culture. I then felt the insignificance of my own life in the scheme of things. While this didn't help my depression much, it did help me step outside of myself and see my life as more than this moment, this month, this year. Things would change, I would learn or move on and go somewhere else. It wasn't the end, just a rock in the road that I needed to circumnavigate in some way. Some sweet, brief peace descended upon me, a levity I hadn't felt in months. I sat there in the shade, sweat trickling down my neck, bugs darting all around, and sighed. It would be okay. Eventually. I had no other option than to move forward, whatever that meant. That's life—moving, growing, hurting, recovering, thinking, feeling. Somehow through it all, I would still be me in the end.

6. *Ground Wires*

I lived with a family in Guatemala for a couple weeks while I studied Spanish and hiked the surrounding lush hills. I visited the white beaches of Nicaragua, Honduras, and Belize. Spent a few days on Isla de Mujeres, explored the pyramids of the Yucatan Peninsula and wove my way through central and northern Mexico.

Still, I was delaying "real life" and the question that came with it: "What am I going to do?"

No closer to an answer, I returned to explore the northwest of the United States, thinking I'd like to move there because I'd never been to that part of the country before. This was around Thanksgiving and Christmas. It was gray, cold and raining just about every day I was there. Being away from family and friends during the holidays is hard enough but, on top of that, I had a growing anxiety about returning to physical therapy. Add the miserable weather and I was pushed down into a hole.

By this time, I'd made it up to Seattle and was staying at a youth hostel. One early morning I woke up and couldn't remember who I was, not even my name. I didn't know where I was. I was in a bunk bed and sensed someone sleeping above me and others in the room. It was still dark. I remained still, trying to think. I lifted my hands to see if they were okay—no marks of damage. I remained still for what I think was an hour. Slowly, my name came back to me. Then I remembered where I was: in a youth hostel in Seattle. I remembered that I had a car. Then I remembered I had a family back east. I could get in my car and drive there. So I got up, found my car and left, driving east.

I didn't turn on the radio. I needed complete silence to orient myself and figure out what I was doing. I could barely drive the speed limit—it just seemed too fast. I thought then that I could find my parents and perhaps even live with them for a couple months. But what good would that do? I would still be me. I would still be in this quandary. And I didn't think I wanted to see the look of concern on their faces or to be asked the inevitable questions about what I planned to do. I was scared, though. This was really rattling me.

I then remembered that a friend of mine, Kristin, was in Denver. I drove to her place and told her I needed help. I just needed to sleep on her couch if I could. She let me stay there for four months. Denver is a bright, beautiful city, full of sunlight. This began lifting me.

I started a routine of stretching each morning and drinking tea—nothing else other than writing in my journal. No plans. Stretching, tea, journal, stretching, tea, journal. That was my day.

Kristin would cook dinner for me when she returned from work. We'd talk and she would just let me be. It was exactly what I needed. I realized, probably much later than I should have, that I needed purpose: to get a job and move out.

I had to do something. I thought that, if I wasn't good enough to be a PT, I at least enjoyed fitness. So I got a job at a prestigious downtown Denver health club and worked at the front desk—I was still too shaken to do anything more involved than that. For six months, I worked behind the front desk, checking people in and handing them towels.

Finally, my manager took me aside. "We hired you because of your PT background and expect you to work at least as a personal trainer. Why don't you get on the stick and start seeing clients?"

So I nervously became a personal trainer. Almost instantly my schedule filled with clients. They all had aches and pains they tried to exercise through. Because I was a PT, could I help them? It was as if there were a legion of walking wounded out there that I just discovered. These people looked healthy and fit but secretly many, so many, had chronic aches and pains. Almost all had been through a host of PTs, chiropractors, massage therapists, and doctors but were left with stubborn pain apparently no one could fix. They all had good insurance and expendable income to work with anyone they wished but, for one reason or another, couldn't find the answers.

They had fallen through the cracks of our medical system. Even in Denver, a fitness-oriented town where there are many elite health professionals, all these people had been unable to find solutions. If the cream of the medical community couldn't help them, then maybe I wasn't so terrible? When I realized this, I let out a deep breath I didn't know I was holding. I suddenly didn't feel so alone.

I had a fundamental belief that pain happened because of how we use our bodies. Much like my toaster or motorcycle, there should be a logic to the connections between function and the structures that are breaking down. But in PT school, I was only taught the separate parts—not how they all fit together from head to toe to create movement. For instance, anatomy class was focused on memorizing origins and insertions of muscles, nerve pathways and how those muscles moved a joint. Even in orthopedics, some of this was put together to demonstrate how it all worked to, say, raise your arm overhead or to walk forward. But there's so much more to it. School taught the basic mechanics of movement but not the significance or repercussions of movement or lack of it.

It was like learning that there's a ground wire in a toaster and how fix it but not about its relationship to the heating coils. Or in the case of my motorcycle carburetor, learning about the pin that guides the floats but not about how that makes the motorcycle move. Much later, I learned that it wasn't just my school that was missing these critical connections.

I realized, at this point, that I had three choices:

1. I could continue on as I was, helping to heal some people but not others.
2. I could quit being a physical therapist and try to reinvent myself.
3. I could try to figure out how it all fit together and become the best physical therapist I could.

Frankly, none of the three appealed to me immediately. The first choice was out of the question. That was why I was stuck in a deep depression in the first place. Choice #2 was not an option, at least not at the time. It had only been a couple years since graduation. If I followed that option, I'd sink into an even greater depression and feel that I'd wasted years and have to start from scratch without an alternative path in mind.

Number three was the only real choice left. But where could I begin to unravel the body's mysteries? Who was I to think that I could even do it? Far smarter people than I apparently either couldn't or didn't see the value in it. Yet this felt like my only real choice.

So I took stock of what I knew for sure. This was basically anatomy and physiology. I no longer had faith in the treatment side of my learning, as it didn't seem to work for me—at least not as well as I thought it should. And if there were so many people who hadn't been helped by doctors or PTs, then it seemed like it wasn't working for others either.

I began observing my clients, but I didn't know what I was

looking for. I simply noticed how they bent down, reached up, or sat. I started to experiment with some half-formed ideas and saw initial positive results.

The standard training states that you must lock your lower back into an arched position when squatting (lifting weights) from the ground, to protect the back. You see this in almost any ergonomic seminar or piece of advice on the Internet. I've even seen a little moving model of this on someone's desk once, where the back is locked while the model squats and stands up.

Yet many of the people I saw with back pain would lie on their back and pull their knees to their chest to ease their pain, rounding the lower back. This is the opposite of that bending advice. Who better to know if something eased their pain than the actual patient? So I began experimenting with allowing people to sit or squat down with a rounded back instead (with light squats only). Most reported that this felt much better for their back. Gradually many felt their pain melt away as they introduced this concept into the rest of their day.

Another personal training dictum was that the knees should not travel over the toes when squatting. I remember a lead trainer running up to me to point out my error when training someone with squats. "Then why are our ankles built to allow this?" I asked her, thinking of my extensive travels in Asia where people had been squatting for thousands of years, allowing their knees to move forward over their toes.

I started paying attention to peoples' shoulders when they lifted weights over their heads. I noticed some peoples' shoulder blades were asymmetrical when doing this. After some queries, I learned that almost all these people had had shoulder surgery at some point. While their surgery arm could reach just as high as the other arm, the shoulder blade acted very differently from one arm to another. I simply tried to get the surgical shoulder blade to move like the non-surgical shoulder blade, which seemed to help.

Definitely no miracles, just small wins. Clients were getting better. Soon I was the busiest personal trainer at the club and held that spot for the next three years, until I left.

Buoyed by my small successes, I drilled down deeper to discover more hidden connections. I began working out of my home, on the side, seeing people privately. I felt guilty charging people for my time. I was just experimenting with ideas, after all. I created a policy in which, if I didn't help someone, they didn't pay. That way I could explore relationships between movement, structure and pain without feeling pressure about how long it took me to figure things out. My wife wasn't happy about it, but I couldn't handle the guilt of someone giving me money when I hadn't helped them.

I remember telling one surgeon with back pain I had helped about my payment policy.

He looked at me and said, "Good PT. Bad businessman." Perhaps, but I felt that this was the right thing to do for me at the time. It was the only thing I could do that would allow me time to explore, without feeling pressure to solve a problem. Along with this approach, I began to feel better, about myself and about my life in general.

I hadn't thrown my education away. Instead, I looked at it through different eyes. I no longer held my instructors' knowledge as gospel. That slight shift in thought set me free.

I then remembered Lois, one of my classmates, talking about Dr. Shirley Sahrmann, a PT and PhD at Washington University in St. Louis. She, I was told, saw injuries and pain differently by connecting movements with pain. I attended Dr. Sahrmann's seminars.

Within the first hour of listening to her, I knew I'd found what I was looking for. It was like coming home after a long, arduous journey. She helped me create a system of evaluation and treatment that connected different parts of the body. I took all her courses. I was *that* student, always in the front row, raising my hand and taking enthusiastic notes.

Adopting Dr. Sahrmann's principles, I found my results with my clients at home became even more dramatic. More people sought me out for help, based on word-of-mouth recommendations. Over that year, my depression dissipated. I felt connected to my work. I stopped feeling that I was a failure and began to think that I was on to something special.

There's a saying that goes "When the student is ready, the teacher will come." The truth of that statement revealed itself by more patients with complex issues starting to show up at my door. Dr. Sahrmann had taught me the mechanics of pain but there was something else that was preventing these new clients from getting better. What I noticed was that, while I could correct the mechanics causing their pain, those mechanics would re-emerge, time after time. It was as if their bodies insisted on assuming these painful positions or habits. It was not conscious. This was something on a different level. There seemed to be an inner driving force creating these patterns of dysfunction that I was trying to correct. It was like rain falling on a windshield. Yes, the wipers would wipe it away but very quickly the rain would accumulate again. I needed to understand where this rain was coming from. My tectonic expectations and judgements were still working on me—I couldn't let it go. I had to figure out what this force was.

I received my answer in a phone call from a stranger who lived halfway across the country.

By this time, I had written my *Fixing You* books to help people solve their own pain. One day I received a call from a woman who was sobbing into the phone. She was wrestling with terrible back pain. She'd read my back pain book but couldn't seem to make it work. She even mentioned suicide. I spoke with her for more than an hour. She calmed down but, in the end, we were no closer to a solution for her. Her problem haunted me over the next month or so. It was similar to what I ran into with these new patients seeking help.

About two months later, out of the blue, I received a call from her again. She had fixed her pain.

"How did you do it?" I asked, dumbstruck.

"Have you ever heard of Hanna Somatics?" she asked. "You have to study this, Rick! It's exactly what I think you're missing. It's what you talk about in your book, but they fix it in a different way. I went to a practitioner and she reduced my pain by 75% in one treatment!"

I couldn't argue with her results. I jumped on the Internet to research Hanna Somatics. I immediately ran into a big problem—no research. My training as a PT dictated that all treatment should be evidence-based, meaning there must be research to support it, ideally published in peer-reviewed journals. But I did not dismiss it simply because it hadn't been researched. After all, much of what I had been doing to help people wasn't found in research. I was wary, but I couldn't get our conversation out of my mind. This just might be what I was looking for to help my more difficult patients. Whatever inner force was causing their bodies to assume these postures and to move in ways that caused pain was the rain, in my analogy. It was the nervous system responding to a problem, whether it be pain, anxiety, or something else. But I'd have to step out of accepted medical paradigm to track it down.

I took the leap and completed the training: nine-day sessions every six months for three years. The information was exactly what I was missing—a method of fixing mechanical problems by changing tension generated by our nervous system. The Hanna Somatics training, while complete, is drawn out and slow. It is designed to train a complete novice to become a very good bodyworker. So there is a broad spectrum of abilities of people who begin the training. Few have the tenacity to stick to it. I nearly quit a few times myself, but I knew that this was information that I needed to master, so I stuck with it. Not many medical professionals, or others, for that matter, will devote that kind of time to learning this system.

It wasn't until the fifth session that I realized that the instructors were trying not only to teach me but to *change* me. To make me into a more holistic practitioner. To be gentler and softer with my patients. To observe more and say less so that I could better perceive the problems my patients were facing.

It worked. It changed me as a practitioner and made me all those things and more. More because, in addition to that, I had other knowledge of which they weren't aware, the biomechanics and pathomechanics of movement that complimented their system so beautifully. When I tried to mention this aspect of pain to the organizers, they were dismissive. I get it. It was *their* system. So I quietly integrated the information myself.

With my new hires at my clinic, I try to pass on these Hanna Somatics principles as much as I can. Some of my associates are more receptive than others. In general, medicine focuses on intelligence as the primary prerequisite for inclusion at schools. But this can lead to excluding the softer characteristics that help people: compassion, caring, listening, gentleness. The Hanna Somatics training recognized this importance, too often overlooked for alpha, book-smart students. For many, me included, it was frustratingly slow—but worth it in the end. Not only for me but for my patients.

I updated my back pain book to reflect this new information. I saw even more success working from my home. My books sold well, and people got better faster than ever. I spoke at conferences, answered emails from readers, and had Skype sessions to help people around the world.

But nagging questions still hung over me. Would this work in a real clinical setting? Could this work for everyone, no matter what condition they had? Was it appropriate for surgical patients as well as those suffering from chronic pain? I had a feeling that the answer was yes, it really would work for all. But my inherent inferiority complex kept questions biting at my heels, questions that another person, endowed with an alpha, extrovert confidence, might not have thought twice about.

Working out of my home, I didn't see the volume or expanse of problems that are seen in a typical clinical setting. I didn't see post-surgical patients, I didn't see normal strains, sprains, broken bones or acute car accidents that are regulars in clinics. My clients' pain was chronic, often decades old. And they were motivated enough to pay cash to see me. That motivation helped them achieve their results.

In a clinic, some people come simply because their doctor told them to, even though they don't believe they can be helped. Some people's visits are limited by insurance restrictions, so they have maybe five visits to solve a 20-year-old problem. Some have just gotten out of surgery and are only coming to you because you're close by and in-network with their insurance. Some injuries are acute, some are chronic. Some are young, some are old. There is a whole spectrum of different types of patients seen in a clinic that accepts insurance as opposed to someone charging cash and working out of their home. I needed to know if this would work with the entire spectrum of problems PTs see in a clinic.

I didn't want to work at someone else's clinic because I knew that I needed to begin at my own pace. Many orthopedic clinics, in order to make ends meet, stack patients. So a PT could be seeing two to five patients at the same time, with an assistant or aide to help them. This maximizes billable time and revenue but is not good for the patient. I had done some temp work for one of these clinics and was constantly frustrated that I couldn't get down to the real problems behind people's pain. My intention was to run a clinic the way I wanted to treat patients, with income as a secondary consideration.

6. Ground Wires

My primary concern was seeing if my approach worked with all populations. Secretly, I'd wanted to own my own PT clinic for years. I thought it would be the pinnacle of my work as a physical therapist. But was I good enough? To even contemplate this was a 180-degree turn from where I was after my first years of practicing PT.

I found a PT about two miles from my home who was selling her small clinic. Would I like to buy it? Yes! After 16 years as a PT, my dream finally came true. I felt that my skills were at the point where I could really make a difference. I was ready to share what I had learned and perhaps even usher in a new way of practicing physical therapy.

It was a beautiful September morning. I had just signed the papers to purchase my new clinic. The keys were in my hand when I got a call from my receptionist—it was my first as a clinic owner. After seeing the caller ID, I thought to myself, "Will it be some difficult PT problem no one could answer?" I hoped so. I'd come so far—I'm ready to tackle the world!

"Is this Rick?" my receptionist said. "We're low on toilet paper. Can you pick some up before you come in?"

≋ 7 ≋

Big Man, Small Car

While in my 20s, living in Boulder and before attending physical therapy school, I volunteered for a Navajo hogan project promoting energy-efficient, solar-powered traditional housing as prototypes for reservations. Hogans were traditional homes of the Navajo. The president of the non-profit was an older Navajo man named Ernie.

Ernie was about 5'6" and in his 60s with long black hair punctuated by gray streaks. He had a perpetually serene expression. He was a friendly man of few words but whose broad face would break into a wide grin at the slightest provocation. His attention was often divided among larger concerns, but for some reason, one day I was lucky enough to be chosen to work with him alone. Our job was to tear down a stone wall dividing two rooms in a hogan to create more open space. I looked forward to spending time with him.

We had few tools to choose from but among them was a large sledgehammer and a smaller hammer. The wooden handles of both were pocked with chips and stains from years of service. I grabbed the sledgehammer, leaving Ernie with the smaller one.

I was younger and enjoyed physical work so immediately I pounded away at the wall with visions of it nearly exploding with the force of my sledge—kind of like the Kool-Aid man crashing through a wall bringing his drink to thirsty kids: "Oh yeah!"

For about 30 minutes I thrashed that wall, sweating and grunting with effort. At the end, I hadn't dislodged one stone—they were apparently set more firmly than I thought. I then looked back at Ernie. With a gentle tap, tap, tap of his hammer, he would loosen one stone, carefully place it on the ground and then begin on his next. He already had a small mound of stones while I had none.

Determined not to let him beat me, I went to work again, flailing

64

away at the stone wall, hitting it right in the center. I pounded with furious energy, breathing hard, hands cramping as I gripped the sledge harder. The shock of each hit reverberated through my body like Wile E. Coyote after he ran into mountain. Twang! Again after 20 minutes of effort, not one stone loosened.

Catching my breath, I then looked back at Ernie, his placid face revealing his enjoyment of the work. Not a drop of sweat on his face. Tap, tap, tap went his small hammer and another stone gently dislodged; it was placed lovingly on the ground. He never looked up at me and seemed almost to be meditating.

I decided to observe him more closely and studied his gentle yet precise technique. I then turned with my sledgehammer, this time choking up on the handle, so my hand was near the head, and I gently tapped at the top layer of the wall. With just a couple taps and almost no effort, my first stone came free. I placed it on the ground and loosed my second stone just as rapidly with almost imperceptible effort. Before long I was enjoying the work in a different way, this time seeing my progress with little effort.

After our wall was finished, Ernie simply smiled at me and took drink of water. It wasn't until more than 20 years later his lesson finally drove home.

<hr />

Steve was a towering, athletic 6'3" tall man in his 40s, with close-cropped salt-and-pepper hair. He was an insurance adjuster who was out in his car most of the day traveling to sites when he wasn't at his desk writing up reports. Other than his height, his most prominent features were the perpetual laugh lines around his mouth and eyes. He had a booming voice and loved cracking jokes.

As Steve complained of chronic low back pain, I watched his laugh lines morph into a worried frown. It wasn't until his pain affected his job that he took it seriously. Each site he visited throughout the day required him to spend more and more time stretching his back. The pain had become worse over these last four weeks, and he finally decided to take action.

One of the most telling pieces of information I gather from patients is how their pain began. This holds clues as to the type of injury at the root of the problem. For instance, an injury that occurred after someone increased their running mileage may have to do with a strength deficit or shoe breakdown. Pain after a fall might indicate a tear or strain that needs to heal.

Steve was no help in this regard. His pain began out of the blue. He hadn't changed the number of hours he spent driving his car or working at his desk. He hadn't changed his exercise routine, diet, shoes or anything else. He was under no new financial or emotional stress. This line of questioning was a dead-end for me. The only thing that was clear was his desire to fix his problem. He recently began losing sleep too.

The next obvious issue was Steve's height. Tall people tend to slouch more so they don't stand out in a crowd. Steve did not slouch when standing but he did when sitting—he couldn't help it. Chairs are typically too short for most tall people. Because of their long legs and minimal space under desks, their knees tend to ride up too high which then tilts the pelvis backward, flattening the spine. While this feels good for most people with back pain, too much of a good thing can be bad. Unlike most people of average height, taller people rarely have an opportunity to get away from that constant flattening.

But Steve told me nothing had changed about his work habits. He drove the same number of hours and sat in the same desk chair as always. So it was unlikely this was the problem.

My examination found several problems that could explain his pain. Steve had flat feet which can affect knee and hip orientation and tight thigh muscles which would tilt his pelvis. One side of his pelvis was higher than the other and one side of his rib cage was lower than the other. His butt muscles didn't work as well as they should. He had poor posture when sitting.

Steve only saw me once a week due to our busy schedules. Undaunted and eager to get better, within three weeks he corrected everything we found wrong. He was an ideal patient who eagerly tackled his rehab homework. We even taped his feet to improve his alignment. I tried every trick I had. Nothing helped, though.

But not only had I not helped Steve, his pain was *exactly* the same as when we began. Like that wall I hammered with Ernie so long ago, I had thrown everything I had at Steve! How could all those corrections amount to nothing? The most obvious answer was they had nothing to do with his pain. Steve began losing faith in me. I saw it in his half-hearted participation with treatment. He was no longer eager. He came more out of habit than anything. Frankly, I was losing confidence too. It made no sense.

⇒⊏ ⇒⊏ ⇒⊏

During my first 20-plus years of practice, I hung my self-worth on the success of my patients. If they didn't get better, I was a failure and miserable. If they did, I was a success and on cloud nine. This led to an endless stomach-churning emotional roller coaster ride for me. Any doctor or therapist will tell you this is a really bad habit. But I couldn't help myself. I felt those old stirrings of failure once more.

Steve's case was like a splinter in my brain I just couldn't reach. What was I missing? Our most recent session left us with no more answers. On that overcast autumn day, he was my last patient and I followed him to the door to wish him a good weekend. My spirits were down but he was kind enough to stay chipper through another failed session.

I stood absently at the glass door and observed him walk away—with perfect balance and symmetry, I might add. Then I watched as he folded his 6'3" frame into his tiny two-door Subaru. It was almost comical. His knees came up on either side of the steering wheel. Then it hit me. I ran out and pounded on his window. He rolled it down.

"Do you have a different car you can drive?" I asked, breathless.

"Yeah, I have an SUV. My father-in-law's been borrowing it since his surgery a couple months ago. He can't bend his knee well," Steve said.

"Your homework is to stop driving this car and drive your SUV until I see you again," I said.

He looked at me quizzically. "Okay, if you say so." I'm sure he thought I was nuts.

Steve came back a week later. "My pain is gone! I haven't had it since I switched cars!" he laughed.

Ernie's lesson then came back to me clearly. I could only smile to myself as Steve walked out of the clinic that final appointment. I finally put words to what Ernie had shown me more than 20 years ago: A small effort directed precisely can have more impact than a big effort aimed broadly.

And my addendum: be more precise with my questions.

8

Naked and Afraid

I walked naked along a busy sidewalk. Sometimes I'd be up on stage with a guitar in front of a crowd only then realizing I couldn't play or sing. One time I was naked there too.

Bad dreams haunted me after my decision. I've always had thin skin, and I knew that if I were attacked, it would devastate me. Did I really have the constitution to put myself out there? I was just a guy working out of his house. What if I actually hurt someone? What if my license were revoked? I spent many sleepless nights leading up to that moment.

Eventually I put my fears aside.

⇒⇐ ⇒⇐ ⇒⇐

After a few years of working as a PT, I discovered workshops put on by Dr. Shirley Sahrmann, a professor of physical therapy at Washington University in St. Louis. With her information, my results got better and better. She helped me make sense of the connections I discovered in my patients.

There was a physical therapist I struck up a friendship with at the seminars and ran into him one day.

"How are you finding the information?" I asked him.

"Oh, I'm just taking bits and pieces," he said. "I'm more of a manual therapist and I don't see a use for a lot of it. I don't think patients will buy into it." A manual therapist is one who typically focuses on joint manipulations like a chiropractor.

"But it works really well," I said. "I'm getting great results. My patients seem to love it."

He shrugged dismissively. With that shrug I realized that Dr. Sahrmann's information was being filtered through therapists who might not embrace it. The full impact of her great work wouldn't be delivered to patients who needed it, many who live in rural communities like the one I grew up and worked in, and may only have access to one or possibly two therapists for help.

This is true of all professions—we tend to apply information that fits our training or personality and discard the rest. Because I had been so unsuccessful as a therapist, I had no allegiance to competing approaches I'd already tried, including manual therapy. They just didn't seem to work well, or at least as well as I thought they should.

I embraced Dr. Sahrmann's philosophy because it worked in the broadest populations and across a wide spectrum of injuries. It combined an understanding of the nuts and bolts of anatomy, neurology and biomechanics with movement habits. It was perfect for me.

Dr. Sahrmann's approach involves assessing movement dysfunctions causing pain. The roots of her brilliant work are in analyzing how the body moves to understand and solve pain. For instance, she came up with the concept of scapular depression as a system of dysfunction stressing the neck and head. I was only beginning to realize how pervasive it was, as well as grasping some of the causes, after attending her seminars. She broke back pain down into three primary patterns of dysfunction: Extension, Flexion and Rotation. This corresponded to what I was discovering with my patients as well, although I hadn't yet thought about rotation problems. She'd mapped out each type of problem and gave legitimacy to my discoveries by explaining why what I'd observed was happening. This helped me embrace what I'd been seeing as real patterns of problems in anyone with pain, not just in my own patients. In essence, her information provided the outline from which I could explore more rapidly and confidently those problems I was seeing and how to solve them. Knowing that she had been researching and experimenting with this information for decades prior to my discoveries helped me feel confident I was on the right track, that I wasn't making this up or that the cases I was solving using this information weren't aberrations.

My advantage at the time was that I worked out of my home and could take more time with people, tumbling down various rabbit holes of dysfunction until I reached an answer or a dead end, and then dive into another. I went further, linking foot, knee, hip and gait dysfunction to each pattern. Eventually I could identify the problematic painful pattern and several causes of it simply by watching someone walk into my home and sit down.

From here I developed a systematic evaluation paradigm testing key issues feeding different patterns of dysfunction. Initially it was full of tests, but I continued chasing down causes of problems, distilling them down to a few simple tests that revealed the chinks in people's systemic and functional armor.

The solutions were prescribing exercises to correct strength or tightness that resulted from poor function. It also required that I teach people how to use their bodies better to reduce strain (you'll see what I mean in the next chapter talking about walking better).

➤← ➤← ➤←

Dr. Sahrmann wrote many research articles and two textbooks but, for some reason, her approach wasn't widely embraced in the physical therapy community. I wasn't about to attempt research of my own. I was just one therapist working out of his home, which made me feel that I was somehow incomplete as a professional. I let these thoughts fester in me for a while.

After a year or two more of using Sahrmann's techniques and unraveling deeper pain patterns, the idea came to me that perhaps I could reach people directly through a self-help book.

That's when I decided to write my first book about neck pain. I had a few "miracle" cures, and while the information was unique, it was also consistent. I helped most clients with neck pain or headaches. They were miracle cures to the patients because they solved chronic problems that they hadn't been able to figure out. They weren't miracles to me because I was gaining a better understanding of how the body works as ever-larger or smaller systems of function. The connections I was discovering, rather than being surprises, started making more sense. They became predictable.

So I buckled down and took the next several months to write my first book, shoot accompanying exercise videos, and hire an editor and illustrator.

Not a day went by in that period when I wasn't plagued with anxieties and doubts. "Who am I to write a book about neck pain? I'm no expert. I'm going to be ripped apart by the medical community. I'll be exposed as a fraud—I'm going to get sued!" I knew I wasn't a fraud, that I was doing my best, but this sort of catastrophic thinking has kept many a well-meaning idea away from those it might help.

I realize now that I was a very anxious person in those days although I never thought of myself like that. I think I was responding to pressure to support my family while discovering a better way to help people and get the word out. I was terrified of getting sued in our litigation-loving society. It was all very scary to me, but I felt it needed to be done. In the end, it turned out that no one really paid attention. All that worry was for naught. No PTs or doctors contacted me to tell me I didn't know what I was talking about. Nobody sued me. My license wasn't revoked.

I sent the book to more than 120 literary agents and publishers over the next few months. I received only one response. This good-hearted editor informed me that, because I don't work with celebrities or professional athletes, I had no basis from which to write a book. Essentially, I lacked a selling point. The content, it seemed, was a distant secondary consideration.

I was so thankful for that response! I'd convinced myself that no one wanted to publish it because the information was bad. Instead, it was simply because there was no marketing potential. This "no" actually propelled me forward. I'd already spent all the time and money to write it, so I might as well keep going.

That's why I decided to self-publish and sell the book on Amazon. Once uploaded, it was buried on page 27 of the search results for "neck pain" books. No one would ever find it. I took small comfort in that. I wouldn't be ridiculed. At least it was done. I could relax and let it go.

Three weeks went by. Then I received an email with the subject line "Your Neck Pain Book."

"Oh my gosh," I thought, "there are a lot of words in this email—this could be bad." Here's what they wrote:

Hello Rick,

...I was able to access the videos and found them extremely helpful. I am so glad I ordered your book. After two and a half years of severe pain on the left side of my head, around my left eye and a weird, extreme feeling of discomfort deep in my nose (a symptom I have not come across despite all my research, doctor's visits, etc.), I read your book, did all four rocking stretches numerous times just this past Wednesday and the hand on head

position, and now Saturday I am on day 4 of living pain free. You have literally given me my life back. I had, in the fall of 2007, been on 3 antibiot-
ics for what was assumed to be a sinus infection, then a negative sinus CT,
visit to an ENT which included scoping up my nose, CT of my brain, an
MRI and MRA of my brain, an MRI of my neck, onto a neurologist, who
insisted I had migraines, despite my telling her it was not a headache I have
but head pain (there is a difference), physical therapy appointments which
caused increased pain due to aggressive massaging of trigger points, many
chiropractic visits, which did offer some relief, 4 months of yoga, and acupuncture, which brings me to Dec. of 2009. I was just this past Monday suffering from depression and despair, thinking that this would be the rest
of my life. I am 52 years old and before this in great health. Yours was the
4th book I have purchased on neck pain, but the only one that even mentioned the scapula and shoulder as being a probable cause. My husband is
so happy that I have found an answer that he has actually mentioned flying
me to Colorado to be seen by you. I anxiously await the film clips that I have
ordered and intend to continue the exercises. I have never written any kind
of testimonial before but felt I needed to express my thanks to you. Your
book has become my bible! Thank you again.

Tears slid down my cheeks. My wife was at work, and I was home
alone with the kids.

"It worked!" I screamed. I danced around. I gave the kids a piece
of candy each. Until that moment, I'd never put myself out there to
publicly fail.

I immediately called my mom and read her the email, choking
up as I did so. She was so happy for me and listened patiently as I
blathered on for the next 20 minutes.

I couldn't believe someone got such quick results with such dramatic debilitating symptoms. I'd certainly seen nothing like those
symptoms in the patients I had treated when I wrote the book. It
made me wonder what was going on with her. Later, I was to suspect
a case of trigeminal neuralgia (the story of Lizzy, told in this book).

Her email lifted an enormous weight off my shoulders. All those
years of failure (or at least what I perceived as failure), experimentation, work, time, cost and worry, those sleepless nights and night-
mares had evaporated because of this woman's words. I thought, at
that moment, that if I never sold another book or helped another person, it was worth it to help her. To change her life through words that
I wrote meant everything to me.

In the end, I think she helped me more than I helped her.

⇒ 9 ⇐

The Case of the Shoulder Problem in Her Foot

In medicine, when someone's gone through a lot of practitioners without relief, they're often thought to be beyond help. Such was Sallie's case.

Past failures don't mean much to me, though. I know the types of treatments others have already tried. It doesn't surprise me that they've failed. I used those same treatment approaches in my first years as a PT which is part of the reason I sank into a depression. Most peoples' injuries have been approached by focusing on the joint or tissue that's painful. Medicine is good at that—isolating a structure that's damaged or irritated. We've got all sorts of sophisticated and expensive scans and tests to find these structural problems. So shoulder pain has been seen as a problem with the shoulder, neck pain is addressed by scrutinizing the neck, back pain blamed on the back. The problem is, if you're looking for a structure to blame pain on, you'll have plenty of opportunity to find it in the body somewhere. We're not perfect. Things break down all the time and we function just fine that way. Many people have disc bulges and even herniations with no pain at all. This is especially the case as we grow older. Blaming pain on a structural problem can be like assuming the heating coils were broken in my childhood toaster. Sometimes this is exactly what the issue is. But I don't believe it until I've had a chance to fix the functional and systemic problems that may be stressing those damaged tissues first.

By systemic, I mean the things that affect other things further away. For instance, if a foot is flat and the arch drops to the ground, the lower leg bone subtly rotates inward, following the foot. Since the

73

lower leg bone includes half of the knee, it then rotates inward too, or at least experiences a force trying to rotate it inward. Since the other half of the knee includes the thigh bone, it also then follows the foot, shin and knee. Everything in the leg has a tendency to roll inward at this point, tumbling like a house of cards.

I've learned the body doesn't really like this kind of inward (internal) rotation. It tends to irritate joints, so now we get tissue irritation in the form of inflamed joints or cartilage breakdown or tears. Following this downward spiral further, the pelvis then experiences this internal rotation force. Over my years of practice, I've teased out the ways the pelvis will react to this phenomenon. For instance, that side of the pelvis can tilt forward, causing a height difference between the two sides. Because it's tilted forward, the back then may compensate by arching backwards, creating excessive unilateral arching on that side of the spine and relative side bending and rotation of the spinal bones. Another response could be that, since the pelvis is rotating forward and down, the waist muscles attaching to the pelvis then try to pull it up, creating tension on that side of the waist contributing, yet again, to a side-bending problem where compression results on that side of the spine. As you can imagine, this pattern is often a cause of sciatic or SI joint pain.

I think of functional issues as slightly different than systemic problems. Functional problems are more about behaviors feeding the systems issues. For instance, in the example above, perhaps all this is happening in part because someone isn't walking properly and therefore not activating their gluteal muscles. The gluteals, among their many functions, rotate the thigh bone outward (external rotation). This can also be thought of as putting the brakes on internal rotation of the thigh bone. If someone is walking correctly, it prevents the thigh bone from rotating inward too much, or at least slows it down a bit. This then prevents the knee from rotating in too much, which prevents the shin bone from rotating in too much. This then unloads the arch of the foot, preventing complete collapse and instead introducing controlled collapse. As you might imagine, this can have enormous ramifications on the tissues at any of these joints. Improving walking patterns is a powerful long-term fix.

Back up at the pelvis, if the butt muscles are activating properly, they also assist in stabilizing the pelvic bone from rotating forward.

In this case, the lower spine no longer has to arch to compensate for this movement, which then eliminates the side bending and rotational forces acting on the spine. The waist muscles can continue their reciprocal contractions because that side isn't trying to hold on to the pelvis for dear life, preventing it from dropping down or rotating forward too much.

You can see that a butterfly's flapping wings really do cause a hurricane in another part of the body. But the converse is true too: let the metaphorical butterfly rest happily on a flower, sipping nectar, and the hurricane melts away.

That's the relationship, in a nutshell, between systemic, functional and structural issues.

The patient perceives these results as miracles—for example, taping a foot arch up and resolving back pain. But like Sherlock Holmes, I've done my homework to understand exactly what the ramifications are to all sorts of idiosyncrasies of the body or behaviors. In that context, they are not miracles to me. The only miracle I'm left with is how rapidly pain melts away when a system and function are restored. It never ceases to amaze me.

It's also so much fun to hear the astonishment in people's voices that it works.

I remember a field of wildflowers I once visited in Utah while camping. I was simply overwhelmed by the beauty spread out before me like a purple ocean. After taking it all in, I scrutinized the area around me more closely and found there were actually small patches where no flowers grew. Closer examination revealed there were other types of flowers and plants interspersed throughout the sea of purple. Finally, I bent down to study a single flower. It took me back to my botany class as an undergraduate at the Ohio State University. I looked at the petal patterns and leaf shapes climbing the stem, and the pistil and stamen of the flower's purple center. Then I compared it to its neighbor to notice small variations between the two apparently identical flowers.

This type of scrutiny involving the whole as well as the parts and their interactions, most closely describes my approach to solving pain. As physical therapists, I think we've done a good job of looking at the parts. It seems we need to study more about how they fit together as a whole. The body is a system. It should be approached as such when the initial foray into dealing with one part at a time does not yield fruit.

━━ ━━ ━━

Sallie had bright blue eyes, a quick wit and big smile. She taught theater for years before retiring. Like my other theater friends, she had an extra volt of electricity to her personality. She practically glowed when she entered the room on this cold November morning.

At our first meeting, I watched Sallie walk toward my table and noticed several issues right off the bat: a pronounced limp with a leaning posture to the left, a left shoulder sitting just a little too low and unnaturally short steps that favored her right leg. They were subtle. Most people wouldn't even notice these things. It's just my job, like a forest ranger spotting a wild animal in the distance no one else can see.

Sallie had several problems consistent with my observations: chronic left shoulder and neck pain and left-sided low back pain for as long as she could remember. She had scoliosis, which was not so unusual given her age of 70. Sallie also had right knee pain which hurt most when walking and gardening—her pleasures in life.

Smiling, Sallie told me that her left shoulder was her top priority. She couldn't lift a bag of groceries without extreme pain. She couldn't get dishes from her cabinet or food from her fridge using that left arm. She had to use her right arm instead, which started to act up too. Her left arm was virtually useless and her back and right knee pain were so severe that she stopped walking and exercising. She lived alone and worried for her future independence. Her ever-present smile faded at this confession. I worried for her too.

Sallie's left shoulder problem was first up to the plate. Starting at her pelvis, I methodically assessed the major bones and muscles to understand what all the players were doing and who was misbehaving. Thankfully, I didn't detect any significant tears or other serious problems. After my examination, I explained to Sallie what I felt the issues were. She listened with polite acceptance and a neutral smile on her face—she'd been through it before.

Skepticism can be a dangerous thing. It goes hand in hand with hopelessness. When we don't have hope and have an abundance of skepticism, we tend not to take action. How can anything change if we don't take action?

I have a unique perspective on how the shoulder and neck function, as we will explore throughout this book. It is linked to my deeper understanding of body systems and how a problem in one area may need to be solved at another. This, added to two specialized techniques, Hanna Somatics and Dr. Sahrmann's approach, make my methodology distinct. My results are very consistent. So much so that, if someone does not respond to my treatment in two to three sessions, I suspect a larger problem, such as a tear. I call tears "structural problems" because they have to do with a breakdown of a physical component of a system, rather than a functional problem that speaks to how that system works.

This is a fundamental concept to this book and to my approach as a medical practitioner. I want to help re-frame the understanding of pain in terms of structural versus functional problems and how functional problems cause structural problems. It's easy to spot a structural problem (tears, disk bulges, arthritis and so on). What people and many medical professionals don't take into account is why those structural problems are occurring. They don't just happen out of the blue—there's a reason. This book is about those reasons that others don't seem to grasp.

So with my toaster analogy, the structural problem was the broken ground wire. No matter how we used the toaster, that ground wire would always be broken and so it would never work. The heating coils weren't really broken; they just appeared to be broken. This represents the systemic problem—a broken ground wire somewhere else causes the heating coil not to work (or, in humans, to be painful). The coils are actually fine. It's the ground wire that's not allowing the heating coils to do their job. That is the structural problem underlying the systemic failure.

The functional problem (or the reason behind the broken ground wire) would be that maybe people slammed the toaster door closed too hard too often, eventually breaking it. Or the toaster was continually jostled because it had to be moved to reach into the cabinet behind it. Functional problems are about how behaviors cause systemic problems and possibly structural problems.

If we don't change *how* we're slamming that door closed or

relocate the toaster to a different part of the kitchen that doesn't require it to be jostled, the ground wire will just break again and again. But if that ground wire isn't repaired, no matter how gently we learn to close the door or wherever we decide to move the toaster, it'll never work. Notice that I'm not even mentioning the coils—because there's nothing wrong with them. That's the relationship between structural, systemic, and functional problems. All are critical in understanding pain. This is the core lesson of this book and of how I teach PT.

I taped Sallie's shoulder blade into a position that would decrease strain to her neck and shoulder. It's the same method I developed to help Debbie with her migraines. The tape gave us a window of opportunity to see how her neck and shoulder would feel given ideal circumstances. Thankfully, Sallie responded rapidly and her left shoulder and neck pain were 80 percent improved in just a few sessions. We simply tinkered with those parts of her shoulder system that weren't working well.

As those improved, we weaned her away from the tape. Given this opportunity to function better, Sallie's body took care of the tissue repair. To me, that's where the magic is. I'm there to help the body realign and then the body handles the rest. The human body is the real hero of this book, and of the story of our lives. It's simply amazing how well designed it is, and how it heals itself when we allow it to.

Slowly, I saw the real Sallie peek out from behind the curtain of her pain. Like a fog had been lifted, she finally shone brightly. Hope was restored. That excitement is the part of my job I love most. Sallie was highly intelligent and caught on right away to how she was going to solve all these problems. I would point out the habits that were breaking down her system and she would fix them. Part of PT is my analysis of what is going wrong. Another part is my manipulation to help fix it. But the third component is teaching the patient how not to revert back to old patterns and how to fix issues themselves through proper movement and exercise.

"Well, since you told me that my shoulder pain was due to my habit of hunching down on that side, I started noticing that I did this when I brush my teeth too. And you know what? I was gardening and started feeling more shoulder pain and thought to myself, 'Now,

Sallie, what are you doing to make that shoulder hurt?' and then I remembered what you said about turning my arm in when I'm reaching, and sure enough...."

Soon she came to the clinic like an eight-year-old at Disneyland, brimming with excitement at the discoveries she'd made. Appointments from this time forward became fun.

My general rule for people who have multiple areas of pain is that we work with one area at a time until it's about 75 percent better. At that point, we know we have a handle on it and can move on to the next area. Otherwise, the benefits of treatment become diluted. This rule is harder to keep than you might imagine because most people want to fix everything at once. For some, it's a struggle to hold back until we reach this milestone.

Sallie was able to control herself and we next addressed her back pain. This time she was enthusiastic at the outset. In about four visits, she was around 85 percent better—she couldn't believe it. Then came her right knee pain, which we were able to improve by about 70 percent in just a few visits as well. This was partly because we needed to address many lower body problems to solve her back pain—so she was already well on her way with regards to her knee pain.

When Sallie came in for her next appointment, I could tell something was on her mind. In spite of our success so far, there was something else—a distant cloud that she could never catch. Sallie finally worked up the courage to tell me her biggest concern.

"I never thought we'd make it this far," she admitted, "and I'm so happy. If we can't do anything else, I'm still so grateful. But I have a problem no one has been able to help me with and, if it's possible, I'd like you to look at it." I could see the reticence on her face: would her request be too much to ask? Have we bumped into the limits of her ability to heal? It was her last hold out to the hope of really getting her life back.

"Well, what is it, Sallie?" I asked. "I'll do my best."

"It's my left foot," she said. "I had surgery on it eight years ago and it's been hurting me ever since. It was painful before but now it's just more painful," she said. "It really hurts to walk."

This came as no surprise, which surprised Sallie. I'd suspected the role of Sallie's foot in all this from the moment I saw her walk in for her first visit. I didn't know the extent of the damage, however. I needed to work through her other problems first before addressing what I felt was the ultimate cause. This gave us a chance to build trust and for me to see how well she would respond to my treatment approach. The more trust she had in me, the longer she would allow me to try to help her. Had we begun with her foot and stumbled with different approaches, she would never have come back for treatment elsewhere.

Sallie's left foot arch had completely collapsed. While I saw that her left foot was a major issue to address when we first met, this was actually the first time I closely examined it, as her upper body and back had kept us busy enough. The keystone of her arch, the large navicular bone, collapsed to the ground with each step. Actually, this isn't completely accurate. To say it collapsed to the ground would indicate that, at some point, it would rise back up. But Sallie's didn't rise up. It just remained down with no spring at all in her foot arch. I had only worked with one other foot like this, with minimal success. Sallie couldn't put her full weight on that foot and whatever weight she did put on it was brief. Imagine walking on a loose bag of 26 potatoes—one for each bone in the foot. It would be very unstable and you'd work twice as hard trying to control it.

The surgery on her left foot many years ago had only made things worse. It gave her foot fewer options to negotiate her root problem, her arch. She didn't have strong enough ligaments to hold it up anymore.

"Sallie, I've been working toward your foot this whole time. I think it's the reason you've been having all this pain. Don't worry, I have some ideas," I said. Secretly, though, I was concerned.

Her whole body slumped in relief at these words. I wasn't aware this had been weighing on her so much these past weeks. I was touched that she trusted me enough to bring up this enormous fear of hers. Sometimes it's easier not to address your fears and keep some little flame of hope flickering deep within than to voice the fear and find there's really no solution after all.

The trail of breadcrumbs from Sallie's foot to her other injuries went something like this: because Sallie's left foot was painful, her left waist and rib cage muscles worked overtime to hike her hip up to unload it. Those muscles then dragged her rib cage down. With the hip held up and the rib cage pulled down, excessive compression on that side of her spine lead to sciatic and low back pain.

9. *The Case of the Shoulder Problem in Her Foot*

The left shoulder blade, which is the foundation for all arm movement, rests on the rib cage and has muscle attachments to the neck and head. Because her left rib cage sat too low, the left shoulder blade followed, disrupting its normal movement. This created pain in her shoulder. Her neck pain resulted from strain of the muscular attachments between her shoulder blade and the neck and head on that side. Of course, the right knee broke down because it carried most of the load, thanks to that useless bag of potatoes she had on her left foot.

When I lay it out like this, it's all very simple. Well, at least it's logical to me, like my toaster on the farm or the carburetor on my motor bike in Australia. Our muscles and bones can be thought of like a Rube Goldberg device—a ball falling into a plastic cup can ultimately light up a Christmas tree at the far end of the room. It all seems haphazard until you take the time to tease out the logical connections along each step of the way. That's what I've been up to these past 25 years.

Yet there's more to it, because nothing in our body works without being told to work. How did the hip

A series of compensations occur throughout the body in response to a foot problem, potentially even affecting the neck and shoulder.

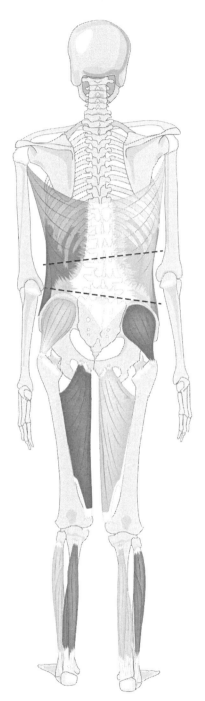

know to lift or the rib cage to depress? How did the right leg know it needed to carry more load? Sallie's brain, of course, is the master controller. And, in her case, it had said, "Oh, now, don't be alarmed by this little obstacle. I'll quietly make this slight modification and we'll both be all right."

But this happened again and again, over a long period of time. Her brain had forgotten its way back to where it had begun, before the problems had come up. It simply adopted this new reality of compensation. These adjustments slipped under her radar while her cerebral cortex, in charge of higher-level executive functioning, worked on daily tasks and goals. What emerged was someone functioning quite differently than the young, athletic teen Sallie once was. The system had shifted to compensate and never shifted back.

Sometimes I feel like a tracker, reading the trail to find where it all began and where it's going. After I explain the trail of cause and effect behind a patient's pain, often I'm met with "I don't know how this happened. I used to be in such good shape when I was younger. I had no idea." Health care professionals can be similarly stumped if they look only at one component of the body at a time, rather than tracking through the system, noting everything that appears off, and tracing the links between errors and inconsistencies, wherever in the body they may appear.

Up to this point, we'd been able to restore better function to all Sallie's problem areas to decrease her pain. But they'd never remain pain-free and working properly if we didn't solve her left foot, which was the root of the collapse of the system—her ground wire.

The best and fastest way to address her foot would be to tape it. Like Sallie's shoulder, tape would give us an idea of how much pain would be relieved if everything were lined up correctly.

A collapsed arch is another matter entirely, though. At the foot, our body weight is multiplied several times with each step. Without an arch to help out, I wasn't sure how she'd respond. The arch in the foot functions like the arch in architecture—it's what holds things up (no wonder you can't spell "architecture" without "arch"). If you want to make a hole in a wall, for a door or a window, you can put in an arch above the opening, like the windows of Romanesque churches. The curve of the arch deflects and disperses the weight and allows for more pressure to be easily withstood. Each time we step onto our foot, the arch of the foot eases the pressure of our weight. Stepping onto a flat foot leads to a world of pain.

Sallie already wore custom shoe inserts made by her podiatrist. However, because she still had pain, I guessed that they weren't as effective as they could be. There are many reasons why inserts might not help people. But through all my experimentation over the years, I've developed a taping technique that works quite well to fix most foot problems associated with a flat arch.

My technique aggressively and precisely lifts the foot arch, holding the ankle in a more ideal position while walking. This is very unlike the taping you see happening on the sidelines for athletes. Tape in those situations is basically creating a snug, slightly mobile cast. That approach is not designed to precisely correct a problem. Instead, it immobilizes a foot and ankle so more damage isn't sustained, and the athlete can continue to play.

By contrast, my technique uses only one piece of tape to offset the spiraling line of force traveling down the leg, collapsing the foot. This single piece of tape allows for maximum mobility while elevating the arch and countering the rotational force traveling through the ankle. While it didn't lift Sallie's arch off the floor, it significantly unloaded the pressure when she walked.

"Okay, try that out, Sallie," I said after taping her foot for the first time.

She got up slowly and tentatively put her left foot down. She focused intently on her pain. Then she took a step with her right foot, weight bearing only briefly on the left, as usual. I worried then that the tape wouldn't help. She stepped with the left foot again and continued walking across the room, slowly.

She limped less with each step.

She turned to face me with tears in her eyes and the brightest wattage smile I'd seen from her yet.

"I have no pain," she said. "I can't believe it! I have no pain."

She still limped, however.

"Why are you still limping, then?" I asked.

She looked at me blankly. "I don't know; it doesn't hurt. I guess just out of habit."

"Then I want you to stop doing that," I said, "or all these problems will keep coming back."

I once had a patient who limped for two years after he had a hip replaced, even though he was pain-free and had the strength not to do so. It was simply the habit he'd formed for the eight prior years of walking with hip pain. He was told by his surgeon to wait until he couldn't stand it any longer to have surgery. But several other secondary problems emerged because of his limping, as in Sallie's case. No amount of nagging on my part could change his habit—only time.

We weren't able to wean her from the tape, though—her foot was too badly changed. The good news is that I use the same approach to cast for shoe inserts—which she loved. Thus the shoe inserts replaced the tape.

When I tape, I manipulate the foot to lift the arch and improve the ankle alignment. I teach my patients to tape themselves or to have a partner tape them. However, if taping seems to be the permanent solution, if the patient can't fix enough other issues to allow us to wean them from the tape, then I recommend that they allow us to cast for shoe inserts. Because we cast for shoe inserts using the same technique we use when we tape, we're confident the shoe insert will work for them. This is important to me because shoe inserts are really expensive, and I see plenty of people who've shelled out lots of money for an insert that either wasn't needed or didn't do the job it was supposed to do.

Many come to our clinic asking for these pricy shoe inserts. Some clinics willingly oblige and just cast them and charge a lot of money. Shoe inserts are high profit centers. I'm always tempted to simply give people what they're asking for—we could certainly use the money. However, it's my responsibility to fix problems if I can, without shoe inserts. In most cases I can, which saves the person a lot of money and leaves them with a new appreciation for how their body works so the problem doesn't come back again.

Now that Sallie could finally walk on her leg without pain, I taught her to walk better.

Walking better is simple but describing walking better is complicated. First, we need to understand why it's important to walk correctly. This is where the butt muscles—the gluteals—come in. The goal of walking better is to naturally turn on and off your butt muscles at the right time and at the right intensity. They are the primary stabilizers of the hip joint. They also help orient the pelvis and lower spine to align them properly. They control rotation of the thigh bone which can affect the knee and shin bone and foot orientation, in terms of deceleration of pronation (flattening of the foot). Finally, proper activation of the gluteals helps relax the waist muscles on the same side of the body.

There is a huge payoff to walking better. In fact, no one leaves our clinic without first learning to walk better if they've been seen for back or any lower body pain. It's that crucial. The most common fault with walking is that of striking the foot on the ground ("foot strike" is how this is referred to in my world), while the pelvis is still behind the foot. Essentially this is a strong heel strike pattern. When the foot strikes the ground in this scenario, the knee tends to lock backward, irritating that small popliteus muscle discussed in Jeni's case. It also means that there is no reason for the butt muscles to turn on, because the foot and knee are absorbing the forces of walking, not the much larger and stronger pelvic muscles.

If you look at the classic Beatles *Abbey Road* album cover, you'll see they're all walking incorrectly. John Lennon, in white at the front, is the one closest to walking well. His pelvis and body are nearly aligned over the advancing foot when it is striking the ground. Paul, George and Ringo's bodies are lagging far behind their advancing foot strike. This is a recipe for damage to any structure in the foot up to the back. Some can get away with it, but those with chronic back and lower body pain cannot.

The waist muscles respond to correct gluteal activation by relatively turning off. If you're walking well and use your hands to squeeze your waist muscles, you'll feel that the muscles on the side bearing your weight will relax relative to the opposite side's waist muscles. This type of relationship happens all over the body. When one muscle group contracts, the opposing muscle group relaxes, to allow supple movement to occur. This at first seems counterintuitive, especially in our physical medicine culture of focusing on strengthening things in order to solve a problem. The body is fluid and needs to relax just as much as it needs to contract in order to move well. This is referred to as "reciprocal inhibition," meaning that the reciprocating muscle group (the one opposite the one you're trying to contract) is inhibited when that contraction occurs. If both groups are contracting on opposite sides of a joint, then excessive tension is delivered to that joint, eventually resulting in a breakdown of structures like cartilage, disks and ligaments. To me this is a beautiful, poetic manner of functioning. In order to move forward, sometimes we have to do less.

In most cases, stability isn't the issue (unless you're a hypermobile person with excessively lax ligaments—a different type of problem). Almost everyone coming to our clinic for low back pain has been told by someone (or some YouTube video) that their core is too weak. As a result, they've done thousands of sit-ups, planks, downward dogs or whatever to strengthen it. Yet they still have back pain. That should tell you, first and foremost, that your core strength isn't actually the problem.

I almost never focus on core strength because that usually isn't the problem. If I do focus on it, I certainly don't assign strengthening exercises to fix it, because those exercises have nothing to do with how that person is using their body. Instead, we teach them to activate the core naturally through changing posture. Correct posture, like walking better, or using your arms better, naturally turns on and off the muscles that should be turning on and off. No one should be walking around constantly tensing their core, or butt, or mid-trapezius—that's unnatural and it doesn't allow for reciprocal inhibition and suppleness of movement.

The combination of taping, shoe inserts and walking better eliminated the rest of Sallie's left shoulder, neck, back and right knee pain. The left foot could carry its own load from now on. The trail I'd followed was no longer there.

Except there was one more thing. A few months later, I caught Sallie limping again.

"Sallie, you're limping again. What's up?" I asked.

"Oh, it's just this callus on the outside of my little toe. It gets really painful. Don't worry, I'm going to the podiatrist to scrape it off today," she said.

"Well, why don't I take a look at it? You haven't mentioned this before," I said.

"Oh, well, that's because every two months for the last eight years, I've just gone to the podiatrist to scrape it off. It heals in a week and then I'm good for another couple months. There's nothing you can do about it. It's just the way it is," she said.

9. The Case of the Shoulder Problem in Her Foot

Nothing gets my hackles up more that someone saying there's nothing I can do about something. I always have to try.

"Let's take a look," I said.

She took off her shoe and sock and there on the outside of her left pinky toe was an enormous red callus.

"I don't remember seeing this before," I said.

"I had it scraped before we started on my foot," she said. "It was better for a while there but it's come back again."

I studied her foot and pulled gently on her little toe, distracting it from her foot. The swollen red callus disappeared and was replaced by a dent.

"Oh, that feels so good!" she said.

I remained there for a couple minutes, tugging on her little toe and moving it gently up and down. I discovered when I moved her toe up, the callus started coming back, but when I moved it down, it disappeared again. I suspected a mechanical cause of this callus.

"Try walking on it now, Sallie," I said

She walked about 20 steps. "No pain," she said, alarmed.

After another 20 steps the pain returned. Because we could interrupt her pain pattern, I felt confident I might be able to solve this last hurdle for Sallie. I asked her to stand in front of me while I observed her foot while weight bearing. The callus gradually returned. But I had discovered earlier that if I moved the toe down, it decreased the callus. I then got an idea.

"Sallie, hand me your left shoe insert," I said. She pulled it out of her shoe and I placed it on the ground and asked her to stand on it. I made a couple marks on her insert where her pinky toe began and ended. I got some scissors, and to her surprise, began cutting away a piece of her orthotic that supported her pinky toe.

"Stand on that, Sallie," I said. She did.

"Wow! That feels good!" she said. "And my callus is gone!"

I then asked her to put it back in her shoe and walk around. She had virtually no pain. I let her walk around for a few minutes.

"Now take off your shoe and sock," I said.

She did and her painful, swollen, red callus was half the size. We were both amazed.

"I'm gonna cancel my podiatry appointment!" she said.

What I think was happening is that there is more than one arch in the foot. There's one that runs side to side as well as front to back. Because Sallie's primary arch had completely collapsed, her big toe was level with or slightly below her pinky toe, upsetting the balance in her front arch. By cutting out a space into which her pinky toe could drop down, we re-established a more normal foot strike pattern between her big toe and pinky toe. This was a completely new concept to me—one that I won't forget. It's thrilling when I discover a new relationship in the body! It's one more piece to our amazing puzzle!

No longer will Sallie need to make visits to her podiatrist or limp.

≡ 10 ≡

Reading Hidden Signals:
Three Pains in the Neck

My sophomore year playing high school football, I began to have frequent "stingers" in my left shoulder. Stingers are the result of a nerve getting pinched or stretched due to poor technique when tackling. These are no fun at all, as any young (or even pro) football player can tell you. They sent electric shocks down my arm. In the last part of our season, the stingers became a normal part of practice and games for me. I figured I'd have to live with them.

We had a weight training system in our basement at our farm that I would use three to four days a week. It was a Universal system, with weight stacks in the center and a bench press and pulleys on the sides. Slowly I lost the ability to hold the handles with my left hand. When bench pressing, I would twist my trunk in order to press weight off my chest on the left side—very bad form. Also while my right biceps could curl 30 pounds, I struggled with five pounds on my left. I could barely lift my left arm above my head.

I tried to ignore it, work around it, and I didn't tell anyone. Not my coaches, not my parents. This was not from some stoic standpoint; I just never thought that it rose to the level of importance to tell anyone. After all, my arm still moved and I had no loss of sensation to my knowledge.

Football merged into wrestling season. I managed to pin a few opponents, but I found that I couldn't use my left arm to leverage any holds or my left hand to grip. Wrestlers would pull my fingers apart as if they were cheap chopsticks. My left arm was only useful as a decoy—it really had no other value on the mat. It wasn't until I was knocked unconscious during a match that my parents realized there

89

was a problem. They had no idea and were properly, grown-up concerned. They took me to a doctor.

"Lift your arms," he said. He placed a hand on each of mine. With a slight touch of his hand, my left arm fell down to my side like a wet noodle. He pressed harder and harder on my right. It didn't budge. I was shocked. I knew it was weak, but this simple test revealed just how weak.

"You've got extensive nerve damage," he said. I wasn't to lift anything, not even my schoolbooks, for the next six to 10 months. My wrestling coach was not happy and made occasional derisive comments. After all, I looked completely normal, especially when I wore a long sleeve shirt to hide my skinny left arm.

The coach was young, and I don't think he knew any better. After all, I wasn't in a cast and had no obvious injury. That's often how injuries went in those days and maybe to some extent today—people have a hard time empathizing with someone if they're not in some kind of cast or don't have a scar to show.

I also wasn't about to quit the team, as I might've lost the varsity letter I had already earned that year. Those were a big deal to me back in those days. So I went to practice every night and matches on weekends.

I was diagnosed at the Cleveland Clinic, which is a prestigious medical center. About a month or so later I was brought in for an EMG study, where they used needles to assess the muscle activity. I remember lying there on the table, the room full of doctors watching me, likely residents in training, observing the treating doctor's technique as he inserted and removed needles from my arms and back. The machine I was hooked up to would make a pulsing sound as it monitored a muscle. A fast, loud pulsing sound rang out when it hit healthy muscles. He demonstrated this on the right side of my upper body. It almost sounded like a race car video game.

Then on to my left side. The pulses were much slower, like someone exhausted slogging through mud. He would put the needle in various muscles throughout my back and left arm and then show the other doctors the same result on the right. They would ask questions I didn't understand.

It was after this test, hearing the differences between the two sides of my body, that I finally believed that something was wrong with me. Before, I hadn't understood the significance of what my doctor was saying. I just knew I was weak. Now I knew there was something broken inside that caused that weakness.

Then, many months later, at the end of my forced non-use period, I went in again for the needle testing. This time, the left was much faster than before and nearly as strong as the right. It was at this point that I could begin exercising again. I was very excited!

The strange thing was that none of this registered in my mind as it was happening. The weakness, the pain during practice, the uselessness of my arm had all happened gradually. I thought I just wasn't strong enough. That I needed to be tougher. That I had to lift more weights and not complain. My body was sending me clear signals I simply wasn't equipped to recognize, much less translate. Even if I had, my naivety might have led me to dismiss them as "to be expected," like the stingers that result from tackling incorrectly. Pain, weakness, and discomfort are not "to be expected." They are signs that something is wrong. My body had been shouting to me, waving for help, but I hadn't noticed or responded.

〓〓〓

Barb was an ER nurse with more than 30 years of experience. She was a no-nonsense, tough woman full of spunk. I could tell she laid down the law wherever she went. She related her story while locking my eyes with her steely blues, willing me to listen. I liked her immediately.

It was late March and Barb's recent bout of neck pain had begun in early February. She'd suffered from chronic headaches and neck pain for years, but it would gradually go away with massage or treatment. In this short interval of time, she'd already been to a chiropractor for several visits, had massage therapy, taken a strong pain reliever—hydrocodone—and tried trigger point injections, where lidocaine is injected into knots of muscles to make them go away. The volume of treatment she'd received in such a short period of time told me that she was in a lot of pain.

She hated to complain and felt that maybe "this ol' cowgirl just needed to pony up and tough it out," as she charmingly phrased it. No, Barb, not if I can help it.

When queried about past injuries, Barb denied ever having had any to speak of. I believed her. She was strong and so full of grit that no injury would dare come near her.

I'll believe my patients until I discover something that doesn't add up with their story—as happened with Barb. Even after I told her that I suspected a shoulder problem as the source of her headaches, she didn't recount the old shoulder pain she'd had 15 years earlier. It was a non-issue to her—she just didn't connect the two. But these old injuries almost always come out in my evaluation or treatment. We bump into a wall and I query the patient about it. Invariably, when I discover something that they hadn't mentioned, I'm met with "Oh, yeah, I forgot about that. It was such a long time ago...."

I remember that I was seeing a gentleman for back pain. He replied that he had no previous injuries. Then, during further questioning, it turned out that he'd played offensive tackle for the Oklahoma Sooners college football team back in the day.

My eyebrows shot up. "And no injuries?"

"Nope," was his response.

Then his wife, sitting beside him, chimed in. "Well, tell him about your surgeries."

He listed several surgeries on his ankles, knees and hips.

"I thought you said you didn't have any injuries," I said.

"Oh, well those are surgeries, they don't count," was his reply.

Once again, this was a reminder for me to ask more specific questions, as in the Big Man in the Little Car story. I need to actively listen but, most importantly, I need to verify, based on my examination.

At our initial evaluation, I determined that Barb's problem came from her shoulders. I treated them, which eliminated her neck pain and even her headaches. I taped her shoulder blades into a better position, just as I'd done with Deb to help with her migraines. I also have a technique where I lift the shoulder blade from the trunk, creating a small gap. Typically, the shoulder blade becomes adhered to the trunk in the case of shoulder injuries, preventing it from moving. Due to its inability to move well, stress then blooms away from this central problem, like dropping paint on a wet piece of paper and watching it bleed.

These two treatments are usually my go-to interventions to test my theory that the shoulder blade is the source of someone's pain.

When it is, in my experience their pain diminishes between 30 and 75 percent after just one treatment. The next question then is "why?" We've determined the systems problem, so now we begin searching for ground wires.

Barb's ground wires were found in her rotator cuff muscles. She was surprised.

"But I don't have shoulder pain," she said.

"That may be, but when I treat your shoulder blade, your headaches and neck pain go away," I replied.

"Well, maybe my shoulder problem is coming from my neck," she countered.

"That's unlikely, Barb. Your neck pain began again just a few weeks ago but the problems I'm seeing in your shoulders are much older than that." She'd had neck pain and headaches for years, on and off. This was just the latest bout.

"How can you tell? Maybe they happened because of my neck," she said, staring me down.

This was a fair question. How could I tell which came first, the chicken or the egg?

When Barb raised her arms up in the air, she sank her shoulder blades down toward her hips and pinched them together, like a dancer or a gymnast. Barb learned this in her yoga classes, which she'd taken for years.

In these classes, it's common to hear an instructor cue attendees to "bring your shoulder blades down and back into your back pockets," "squeeze your shoulder blades together" or "lengthen your neck" when raising your arms into the air. This is one of my biggest pet peeves of dysfunctional movement that's taught in exercise classes. It's a shorthand mantra called out in class by an instructor, and it can lead to damaging habits if incorrectly interpreted or implied beyond the boundaries of a yoga or Pilates series.

This isn't just taught in yoga classes. It happens in Pilates, dance and gymnastics too. The desire to create a long neck, which is aesthetically pleasing, is the core of the problem. People are ruining their shoulders and their neck to achieve this.

Creating a "long neck" is the opposite of proper shoulder blade function. Without going into all the biometric markers, the shoulder blades' general role is to rotate outward and lift as the arms move away from the body. This helps the shoulder muscles do their job: to lift the arm. Lifting the arms while creating a long neck essentially short circuits this whole process (to maintain our toaster analogy). Shoulder blade rotation and lifting also maintain a proper length and tension in the muscles connecting into the neck from the shoulder blades.

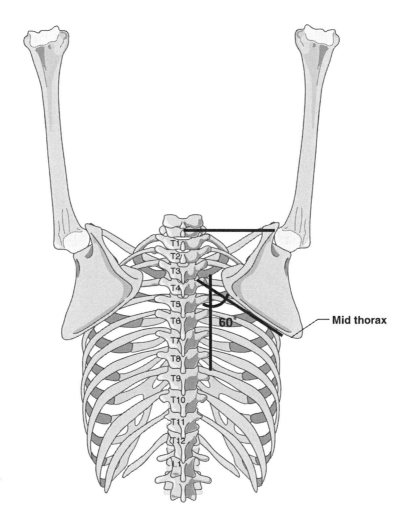

The shoulder blade's role is to assist with overhead motions and has specific landmarks to measure its function.

Barb was such an adept yoga practitioner that her critical shoulder blade muscles were turned off as a result. It took a bit of training to turn off these muscles so completely. Certainly more than a month. She had essentially trained, over an extended period of time, her shoulder blade muscles to no longer do what they were made for. The fact that Barb couldn't even activate them at all told me this was an old problem.

When basic rules of proper movement are broken, pain results. Like tackling with poor form in high school caused my pinched nerve. In Barb's case, the small muscles linking her shoulder blades to her neck became strained as a result of her habit of pushing her shoulder blades down toward her hips. Judging by her personality, Barb probably made it a point to beat everyone in the yoga room at it too.

I explained this to Barb and added, "If these were recent changes then you'd be telling me about shoulder problems too. But you haven't mentioned anything about your shoulders."

"That's because they don't hurt," she said.

I smiled. We went back and forth like this for some time. Some practitioners don't like to be challenged in this way, but I don't mind. It's actually kind of fun for me and can expose faults in my thinking or perhaps problems I hadn't considered. I was pretty sure about Barb, though—I'd seen this many times before.

Because yoga is an ancient movement art, the assumption is that it must be good for you. In most cases it is—except when it isn't. You need to remember that, hundreds of years ago, people didn't know about femoral anteversion or retroversion. They didn't understand how the gluteals control femoral rotation or the tracking of the hip joint in the socket. They didn't know that there were shoulder blade biometrics or what ideal movement was. Yoga was created out of the best information available at the time. But sometimes information needs to be updated. Just because your body *can* do something doesn't mean it *should* do something.

Sometimes, depending on what's wrong with you, yoga will not be the right solution and may even hurt you more, as in Lizzy's case in the next chapter.

I've noticed, over the years, that flexible people gravitate to exercise that rewards flexibility. They think they need more flexibility to solve their pain and typically avoid strengthening. Strong people tend to gravitate toward strengthening to solve their pain and they therefore avoid lengthening. We don't like to do things we're not good at. But sometimes when you find something you're not good at, it may be exactly what you need to be doing. On the other hand, there may be a very good reason why you're not good at it—because you shouldn't be doing it. That's where the value of seeing a physical therapist comes in: to evaluate your body, especially in relation to a desired activity. We can show you what might go wrong and how to make your mechanics better to avoid injuries.

But Barb's defensiveness didn't come from a conviction that yoga is a panacea. Barb was an old school emergency room nurse. She'd seen it all. She wasn't about to believe some story a random PT was telling her—especially after so many other failed treatments in the past. Even my attempts to show her how fixing the shoulder blade would fix her headaches didn't pass muster with her.

What I was saying was contrary to popular medical wisdom. Current wisdom is that all problems in the neck and head emanate from the neck, not the shoulder. This is because the nerves that feed our upper body system emanate from the neck, and so it follows that all problems must stem from this—except that it doesn't. That's too simplistic a way of seeing the body. In fact, the upper body system puts a strain on the neck, which then can feed back down into the upper body system. It's a negative loop.

Barb had never heard of such a thing. Her doctors had never heard of such a thing. And probably most impactful, in the era of Dr. Google, the Internet had never heard of such a thing. There's an assumption that Google will reveal all—if there's a treatment that hasn't been published extensively online, patients look upon it with suspicion.

But Barb was stubborn and wasn't about to have anyone pull a fast one on her. After all, no one had even looked at her shoulders before. She was a nurse who'd seen it all.

She insisted on a neck MRI.

"That's fine, Barb," I said. "Just know that many changes you might see on your MRI are normal and happen with age. They often have nothing to do with pain."

As we age, our spines naturally develop signs of wear and tear, like disc bulges, arthritic changes, thinning of the discs between vertebrae, even small fractures. These changes become less significant as we age because they are the simple result of normal wear and tear. Most people with these types of changes have no pain at all.

Barb's MRI revealed minor bulges in her discs and small arthritic changes too. Frankly, it wasn't very impressive—I'd seen far worse MRIs in people with less pain than Barb. Also, small world department, I noticed the name of her doctor. I happened to be treating him for a hip problem.

"I went to a neurologist with my MRI," she said a week later, when she came to the office. "He said there's no medical evidence supporting the shoulders creating neck pain."

"Yup," I said, "he's absolutely right. But let me ask you this, Barb. If your shoulders have nothing to do with your neck pain, then why is the neck pain relieved when we tape your shoulders?"

That stumped her for the time being. I used this opportunity to convince her to get a shoulder MRI. I wanted one because her pain would not decrease without the tape. Usually, after a week or two, people can fix their strength and range of motion problems and then wean off the tape. Not Barb. I was concerned that there was something more serious going on that I'd missed earlier.

She rolled her eyes. "Okay, I'll get a shoulder MRI."

Since her doctor knew me, and was my patient, he was not disarmed by my request for an MRI that seemed to have nothing to do with anything relevant.

The results shocked us all.

Barb had full-thickness rotator cuff tears in *both* shoulders! This means that the primary rotator cuff muscle was completely detached. On both sides.

When her doctor came to my clinic for his next visit, to work on his hip, he immediately brought up Barb's MRI. "I've never seen anything like this!" he said. "I'd never think to even look at her shoulders. How did you know?" I explained the connections and showed him a simple test I'd devised to figure it out.

I hadn't found Barb's rotator cuff tears in my earlier testing. This was likely because she was so good at compensating with her neck. Even after discovering the rotator cuff tears, I tested them

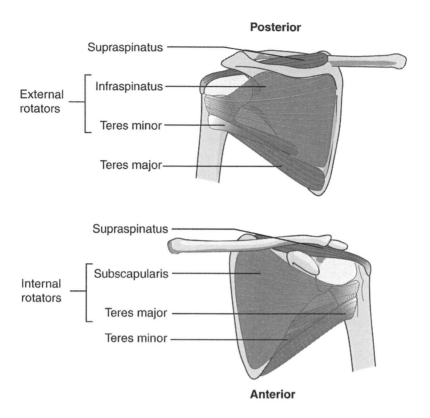

The most common rotator cuff muscle torn is the supraspinatus, which is responsible for assisting with raising the arm.

again. This time I saw how she did it. While her shoulder blade muscles were incapable of anything, she recruited her neck muscles and her shoulder muscles to compensate. This must've taken years to master.

"I thought you said you never had an injury to your upper body before," I asked her, mock-accusingly.

"Well, now that you mention it," she replied sheepishly, "I did hurt my shoulders about 15 years ago. This cowgirl just ponied up and, after a few weeks, the pain went away. I never thought about it again. By the way, my shoulder surgeon said there are no studies connecting shoulder problems to neck pain or headaches."

I smiled. "He's absolutely right, Barb. There aren't." But I think she was coming around to my way of thinking.

The only way to prove my theory correct was if Barb had rotator cuff surgery to repair the torn muscles. We were out of other options. Treating her shoulder blades eliminated her headaches. When we stopped, the headaches would resume.

The rotator cuff muscles, in this example, were the ground wires affecting the system. The headaches were the heating coils—the manifestation of something wrong with the system. The functional cause was likely her manner of using her arms that promoted scapular depression: postural cues to pinch the shoulder blades together and squeeze them down to create an erect spine. Over the years, this shut down her scapular positioning muscles, the trapezius and the serratus anterior. Sometimes when muscles shut down, they become neurologically weak, as in the mid-trapezius. This means the muscle isn't truly weak; it's just that the brain has forgotten how to engage the muscle well. This also happens to the glutcals with poor walking habits.

The serratus anterior is a weird muscle that begins in the side of the rib cage toward the front along many rib levels and inserts along the medial border of the shoulder blade (the flat border closest to the spine). This muscle is interesting in that, in the presence of anxiety, stress, or injury, it tends to contract, locking the shoulder blade to the thorax. I believe it's part of a larger pattern of muscles contributing to another deep reflex pattern, the startle reflex, which I learned about in Hanna Somatics training. That's another hard-wired reflex pattern we're born with.

You can watch YouTube videos of babies being startled and see the same pattern response. Typically, the arms come in, the shoulders shrug up and the eyes blink firmly. I think that the serratus anterior is responsible for the portion of the behavior involving the arms pulling in toward the body. I've found that, in order to separate the shoulder blade from the trunk, I need to relax the serratus anterior muscles with a gentle technique, getting them to let go of the shoulder blade.

The question of which muscles were locking the shoulder blade to the trunk stumped me for years. I thought it was the trapezius in the back. But a local PT graduate program, Regis University, opened up their cadaver lab to PTs interested in refreshing their anatomical knowledge. I jumped at the chance. I had so many questions about what I had seen clinically over the years. Because the university was using these cadavers for their PT program, they were already dissected to varying degrees. To test my particular question of which muscles were adhering the shoulder blade to the trunk, I needed to find a couple of cadavers whose shoulder blades had not been completely removed. There were a few.

While other PTs poked, prodded and observed, I sought out these cadavers, gently rolled them onto their sides and began mobilizing their shoulder blades, just like I did in the clinic. Holding the shoulder blade away from the body, I traced the muscles to see which had become taut. To my surprise, it was the serratus anterior, which I hadn't even considered before, due to its strange orientation.

Once I confirmed this with the other cadavers' shoulder blades, I sat at home thinking about this. If the serratus anterior are locking down the shoulder blade, what would be the best way to get them to let go? I studied the architecture of the muscle. It was thin and broad and lay right over those sensitive ribs. Whatever I would try, it would need to be gentle. I then reached to my own serratus anterior and experimented with different types of touch. I quickly settled on a broad palm technique that felt soothing.

I began experimenting with this technique with my shoulder blade patients and found it very quickly unlocked the shoulder blade from the trunk. I now alternate between this gentle massage and lifting the shoulder blade to release the blade from the trunk. I've also found significant trigger points in the serratus anterior that refer pain into the neck, head, face and hands. There are no direct anatomical connections to explain this. Instead I choose to think of it as massaging the center of a spider web of various tissues, which results in all points responding to that central massage.

After several more months of thinking about it, Barb eventually relented and had the surgery. Her neck pain and headaches disappeared and never returned—at least on that side. But rotator cuff surgery recovery is long and painful, so she only repaired one side at a time. We chose the side where her headaches were worst first. Later, she repaired the other rotator cuff. One of my other therapists worked with her post-surgery, but I would check in time to time to see how she was. To my knowledge, she hasn't had a headache since, or if so, they were a shadow of what they once were.

Shortly after I started with Barb, Sharon came to the clinic after enduring chronic neck pain and migraines on both sides of her head for many years. Like many patients who end up at our clinic, she had been through a lot of other practitioners. Often these people fall off their doctors' radar because they seek alternative care like chiropractic, massage, acupuncture, diet, etc. This can go on for years before they finally come back to their doctor again. I think this is how it was with Sharon. Her doctor had just recently learned of our clinic and sent her over. Sharon's right side was worse than her left, and when she was in pain, it was difficult for her to even lift her head to look up.

She had occasional numbness or tingling in her hands, which told me that the nerves in her neck were getting pinched. Her arms felt weak. She'd seen a chiropractor and massage therapist for years and decided to try something new. She couldn't remember any particular incident that marked the beginning of her problem.

Sharon was a young, athletic woman in her mid–30s who played softball, played cymbals in a band, took guitar lessons and worked in IT. Whenever anyone tells me they're in IT, my eyes glaze over. I'm mechanically inclined, which means I'm digitally declined: computer programming just seems about as tenable as shaping a soap bubble.

My examination found issues similar to Barb's. We set about strengthening Sharon's mid-trapezius muscle. This muscle is key in gaining control of the shoulder blade. Through the years, I've settled on a very precise technique to activate it properly. My strengthening is not like that of a typical PT. I don't begin with the classic rotator cuff strengthening exercises that are ubiquitous in shoulder rehab. Typically, with chronic shoulder problems, the middle portion of the trapezius has grown weak, so that's where I begin. I use just one strengthening exercise. Just like that Native American story of a well-placed focus is better than a broad-based effort. It seems to be key to long-term shoulder girdle strength and health, which means it's also key to the health of the entire upper body system. I also taped her shoulder blades to compensate for the weak trapezius, as I had with Barb.

We tried dry needling as well, using acupuncture needles to release key spasmed muscles. Dry needling is a physical therapist's application of acupuncture needles. If you've ever seen a picture of a person's body as understood by traditional Chinese medicine, you'll see that the body has lines that intersect all over it, like a grid. These are meridian lines which correspond to energy flow between different organs and parts of the body. An acupuncturist applies their needles according to this map. The system allows for what I've found to be true throughout my career: that points far away from a problem may have a relationship to the actual problem. This is similar to my thinking, but traditional Chinese medicine takes it much further, suggesting that acupuncture not only affects different parts of the musculoskeletal system but also internal functions, too, like digestion, breathing and the heart.

Dry needling uses acupuncture needles in muscles from which we would like to release pain-causing tension. There may be overlaps between the two systems, but the intent is very different. Applying the needles actually reduces reflexive spasms in the muscles. If you understand which muscles are in spasm and causing pain, dry needling can be very effective. But it's important not to forget to solve the "why," the reason a patient is in spasm. Once again, medicine is good at identifying a problematic tissue but not so good at identifying why that tissue is problematic.

Within a few weeks, Sharon's left neck pain vanished. That was the good news. The bad news was that her right neck pain remained.

I was suspicious.

Sharon's right neck and shoulder pain could disappear, too, but only when she wore the tape—like Barb. Once the tape was removed, her pain would swiftly return. It also rang alarm bells when we found that dry needling resulted in a heavy achy feeling in her arm the next day. This is not expected of healthy tissue. I've learned over the years that this likely indicates a tear or some other tissue damage. We continued trying to help her right shoulder but I'm ashamed to admit that her pain got worse. This was yet another red flag for me.

"I never noticed my shoulder pain until you started treating it," she said.

That didn't make me feel very good. But there was clearly a serious problem happening with her shoulder.

Finally, after a lot of back and forth, Sharon agreed to get an MRI. Shockingly for both of us, it came back normal. In fact, it was one of the cleanest MRIs I'd ever seen. A pristine shoulder. Some MRIs are more powerful than others. A 3T MRI is the most powerful on the market. The most common is the 1.5T, so the 3T is twice as powerful ... but also a lot more expensive. Most things show up well on a 1.5T, so most clinics use them. I think Sharon's MRI was a 1.5T. Also she did not use a dye contrast which exposes tears in tissues. Some surgeons, though, only trust 3T MRIs to get more detail—a 3T would likely have shown the issue.

MRIs also do less well with more chronic conditions, as scarring may obscure the actual tear. Finally, the shoulder is a complicated structure to image. The labrum is even more so, as it can be partially hidden deep in the shoulder socket. It's not uncommon for an MRI report to show that someone has a rotator cuff tear, only to find after the surgeon goes in that there are several other problems it didn't detect, like small tears in the labrum or biceps or other rotator cuff muscles, among other things. Whatever the reason, Sharon's MRI came out clean. Based on these results, her shoulder surgeon recommended she see a pain specialist. He also said that her shoulder probably had nothing to do with her neck pain or migraines.

I was upset about this recommendation. A pain specialist is primarily interested in controlling pain through medications or cortisone shots. Sharon was young and athletic. I refused to believe there was nothing wrong with her shoulder, which seemed to me to be at the heart of her neck pain. It didn't add up.

I sent her to another shoulder surgeon for a second opinion. He told her that if she didn't feel better after six more weeks of conservative care, he would perform exploratory surgery on her shoulder. We had worked with this surgeon before and he trusted our judgment. Six weeks passed and she went into surgery. She emailed me a week later to tell me that her doctor had repaired two massive labral tears in her right shoulder—the largest labral tears he had repaired to date.

The *labrum* is a piece of cartilage that surrounds the shoulder socket and deepens it, allowing the head of the arm bone to sit more securely in the socket. It also creates a vacuum within the socket and this suction helps hold the arm bone in place. With a torn labrum, this vacuum is disrupted, and the arm bone loses that nice secure fit into the shoulder socket.

Almost immediately after Sharon's surgery, her neck pain and migraines disappeared. Even through her rehab, she had no pain other than that associated with her surgery.

━ ━ ━

Around the time Barb had her neck MRI, Alex came in for his chronic left-sided neck pain. He'd read my book and, with a little searching, found I lived near him in Denver.

Alex was 6'3" and built like a linebacker—I'm sure any NFL team would drool over him. He was solid muscle, weighing in at around 240 pounds. He practically filled the room.

Alex reported that, two or three years earlier, he'd had a mild left shoulder acromioclavicular (AC) separation. The *acromion* is a bony part of the shoulder blade which then connects to the collar bone (the clavicle), the junction of which, the AC joint, is held together by ligaments. The clavicle then articulates with the central bone of the rib cage in the front—the sternum.

The sternum is the only bony connection of the shoulder system to the trunk of our body. Essentially our shoulders and arms are floating objects. So a separation of the AC joint disrupts this already tenuous communication with our trunk.

Alex also admitted that he probably had some labral tears in both shoulders. Remember that the labrum is what Sharon had wrong with her right shoulder. Looking at his muscle bulk, I guessed there was more to the picture than he'd painted. You don't get that big and strong without damaging something. Alex worked out constantly and ignored these minor issues, which would be major to other people.

After he shared his history, we then went through our examination, from which I noted two significant findings. The first was that he had extraordinary range of motion in his shoulders. Usually with very muscular people comes a degree of tightness in the muscles. Exceptions to this rule are gymnasts, baseball pitchers and swimmers. Alex was none of these.

While having excessive range of motion is a blessing if you're involved in any of those sports, for ordinary people, too much motion can cause wear and tear in a joint. Because of this general looseness and his labral tears, I imagined Alex's shoulder joint was like a washing machine that was out of balance, careening off the sides of his socket. Unlike a washing machine, though, he didn't have an automatic shut-off when the system got out of control. He continued lifting high repetitions of very heavy weights. My general rule of thumb for heavy weightlifters is that those aches and pains are real and they add up. Get them checked out by a physician or a PT so you at least understand what you're ignoring.

In general, there is also a carryover for the range of motion you are strengthening. Most people don't need to strengthen the full range of motion to become strong through the full range of motion. I recommend strengthening through about 75 percent of your available range of motion. That last 25 percent or so that you're loading through is typically where damage is done to the tendons, ligaments or joint surfaces. While the body is made to go through that full range of motion, it's not made to do so under heavy loads repeatedly—something will eventually give. Better to avoid it all together.

Part of my exam involved testing strength. When I tested Alex, it was like that scene in *Rocky IV* when Apollo Creed is about to fight Drago, the Russian boxer. They bumped fists before the fight, but Drago's fists were like unyielding steel. Apollo's normally easy smile flickered briefly. *I'm going up against him.* I'm testing all the major muscles for weaknesses. I couldn't make him budge with any of the tests. Like the doctor did with me, testing my shoulder strength by having me hold both arms straight in front of me, then pressing down on my right (it didn't budge), then on my left (which collapsed immediately). It was like this with Alex, minus the collapsing—just unyielding strength, even as I increased the load to test for pain.

This was my experience with all of Alex's testing, except for one key muscle group that happens to be involved in stabilizing all shoulder and arm movements—the mid-*trapezius* muscle I mentioned in Sharon's case.

The trapezius is amazing in both its architecture and function. It's a very large, broad muscle that runs from the base of the skull down to the lower back bones of the thoracic spine, where the ribs attach. It then connects to the shoulder blade and collar bone. It's so big that we divide it into three zones when considering it, upper, mid, and lower, each of which has their own job to do.

With weightlifters like Alex, you tend to see bulging, over-developed upper trapezius muscles, which give the appearance of a thick neck. Alex's lower trapezius muscles were also incredibly strong, from all his lat pulldowns to create that classic V-shaped torso found in bodybuilders.

The mid-trapezius muscle is critical to proper shoulder blade strength and control. Alex could barely lift his arm against gravity on his left side during my testing. He was shocked to find a chink in his armor. He hadn't realized that he could possibly be so weak, especially with all his usual strength training targeting his back muscles. I'd found the same weakness with Barb and Sharon.

To his credit, Alex attacked his one weakness as if it were a personal affront. Strengthening that portion of his trapezius, together with my shoulder blade taping technique and a little bit of dry needling in his shoulder, completely eliminated his neck pain within a few weeks.

But then it returned again and again. Just like Barb and Sharon.

I asked Alex to get an MRI and see a shoulder surgeon. His MRI showed a variety of issues, including labral fraying, small tears in two rotator cuff muscles and scarring of a shoulder ligament.

Rotator cuff muscles are a group of muscles that create precision of the shoulder movements. Tears indicate the potential for larger problems. His shoulder surgeon wasn't concerned about any of this and did not recommend surgery to fix them. In my opinion, he was just looking at the shoulder as a shoulder—that's his training. He didn't understand that this was affecting Alex's neck. Also, because Alex was so incredibly strong, there was no reason to repair these apparently small issues because there was no functional breakdown in Alex's system. Lastly, partial rotator cuff tears can heal on their own, so I'm guessing that's what the surgeon was thinking. I didn't think this was likely, however, because of how much and how often Alex challenged his muscles with weight training. But the bottom line was, at least from the surgeon's point of view, Alex was functioning not only well but superiorly, so why operate?

Alex's issues concerned me, though, given the volume of his weight training and persistent pain. While any one of these findings may not raise a red flag, the spectrum of tissues showing damage indicated to me that his shoulder was in the process of breaking down. Alex needed as much stabilization as possible for that shoulder because he wasn't about to stop weight training—it was clearly his passion.

Alex asked his surgeon if the problems found in his MRI could lead to his neck pain.

"Highly unlikely," was the surgeon's brief response. But Alex asked him for a cortisone shot to the shoulder anyway.

Cortisone is a steroid that shrinks irritated tissue, calming it down. Often, it's accompanied by lidocaine, which numbs the area. Alex's shot to his shoulder completely cleared up his neck pain for several weeks. This confirmed to us that his shoulder was the true culprit behind his neck pain.

The doctor also gave Alex a set of simple rotator cuff strengthening exercises which, together with a few others, resolved Alex's neck pain as long as he continued them. I'd neglected to give Alex these basic exercises because he tested so strong initially. However, had I repeatedly challenged these muscles, I likely would have found that they had little endurance and needed some attention. I kicked myself for missing that.

Alex opted for strengthening his way to recovery. This played very well into his strengths (literally)—weight training. We stayed in touch via email over the next several months. He had few to no symptoms after the shot and strengthening plan. But I fretted over the long-term damage that might be happening to his shoulders.

These three stories of pains in the neck and headaches that were actually shoulder problems in disguise clearly show the connection between shoulder function and neck or head pain—the ground wires. I could relate many, many more. There are other connections in the body that are largely unknown to the medical community because they cannot be isolated in medical studies.

Why not? Our bodies' complexity of movement does not lend itself to double-blind studies—the gold standard for inclusivity in medical studies. At best, these stories would warrant a case study which has the lowest validity in the spectrum of research, and so are often ignored.

I don't fault surgeons for not knowing of these connections. Their training is focused on being the best surgeons they can be. This knowledge doesn't help them in that regard. Just as I don't read research on current surgical techniques. It's not pertinent to my success as a PT.

I suppose this really speaks to the specificity of medicine. After all, you wouldn't ask a cardiologist about a urinary tract infection. It's just not their specialty. This places a burden on the patient to understand who to ask for direction. Our body is trying to tell us something. But instead of it screaming out specific instructions, it sends coded signals that we medical professionals have to learn how to read.

⟫ 11 ⟪

Pain Is a Sandcastle

"It feels like a hook is in the left side of my mouth, pulling my lips to my ear," Lizzy offered softly, "and I feel like I have broken glass in my nose."

Lizzy was a 54-year-old mountain biker, runner, hiker, skier—all the typical sports we see here in Colorado. She was active and full of energy.

At least, that's how she should have been. The woman sitting in my office did not match that description. Speaking in a whisper and hunched over, she complained of left-sided head pain. But this was not a headache. It was stranger and more frightening. The muscles throughout her face, around her ear, eye socket, teeth, palate, jaw and the back of her head all hurt terribly.

She was highly sensitive to light and wore sunglasses even indoors. To accommodate, I shut off the overhead lights in the clinic. Sounds above a whisper grated on her and she complained of constant dizziness and nausea. These might have been signs of migraine, but the other symptoms suggested otherwise. Her sense of taste had been altered—she no longer enjoyed food. That wasn't a normal accompaniment of migraines. I couldn't imagine how miserable she must be.

She took medications every 30 minutes to keep her pain tolerable. But Lizzy didn't want to control it; she wanted to get rid of it. She was a photographer and these drugs interfered with her work, her life, and her well-being. She had already been to a slew of doctors and was desperate for help. Her doctor sent her to my clinic after another doctor in his practice had mentioned the good results I'd achieved for another patient. He figured he'd give me a try.

Her symptoms had been relentless for the several months since she'd attended a yoga class. The pain was constant in her jaw and face and spread to the other areas of her head too. She had to lie "just so" in order to finally fall asleep each night and would often wake from pain after just an hour or two. She was always tired. Sometimes she would have to wear a mask to keep breezes from touching her face, as even that would send her into waves of agony.

If this weren't enough, Lizzy's past history involved several car accidents, dating far back to her childhood, which left her with chronic migraines and general neck stiffness and pain. She told me that, since those accidents, she never liked having both arms raised over her head (which made me wonder at her enthusiasm for yoga). Several years earlier, she'd suffered a traumatic blow to her left shoulder which had dislocated it. It was "put back in" at the ER with no further treatment.

Contrary to Mel Gibson's portrayal of resetting a dislocated shoulder in *Lethal Weapon* by smashing it against a wall or pole, resetting a dislocated shoulder is not a violent procedure. Actually, it's quite gentle, involving supporting the arm and gently massaging the upper trapezius and deltoid until the head of the shoulder joint slips back into place—the Cunningham Technique. No pops, no cracks, no grunts. In fact, many people aren't even aware it's been relocated. The arm is then put in a sling with the hand resting near the belly to keep the system stable. There is a capsule that surrounds the shoulder joint to keep it in place. Repeated dislocations mean these tissues are likely becoming compromised.

Though it may sound strange, I was comforted after hearing Lizzy's history, fraught with traumas though it was, because there were clues in it that I might be able to help her. In fact, despite never having treated trigeminal neuralgia before, and knowing of its reputation for never going away, I was quite confident that I understood what was happening to her. I was excited to begin.

The consensus at the time I saw Lizzy was that she suffered from *trigeminal neuralgia* which was thought to be caused by a problem with the jaw. Today researchers have identified that the trigeminal nerve can get impinged by a blood vessel in the brain. This is a structural explanation. A ground wire is good, but my work focuses on the functional causes of pain, the reasons those ground wires are broken.

I had never seen a patient with trigeminal neuralgia before, much less encountered symptoms as severe as these. The trigeminal nerve is a cranial nerve, meaning that it originates in the brainstem, within the skull. Its tendrils reach into the eye sockets, sinuses and mouth. It's a sensory nerve, so it carries information, like temperature and pressure, from the face to the brain. This is distinct from a motor nerve that carries information from the brain to the facial muscles, to make them smile or wink an eye. Until that point, I was used to working with just about anything from head to toe. But I never thought I would actually work inside someone's brain.

During our evaluation, I found that I could press anywhere on Lizzy's left arm or hand and elicit pain in her face and head. This was news to her—no one had ever looked at this before. We also discovered that touching her right arm referred pain to her left face, also a surprise. Past evaluators had only looked at her neck and head, since that's where her pain was. This was mostly due to the belief that trigeminal neuralgia is solely a problem with a blood vessel in the skull. In their thinking, there's no reason to look elsewhere.

I approached her body as a network with triggers sometimes far from the pain itself. Additionally, I found that her left shoulder blade wasn't resting or moving correctly—no doubt from the shoulder dislocation years ago. Her trigeminal neuralgia pain was primarily on the left side of her head. To me, this was no coincidence. To someone who doesn't understand how the upper body system affects neck or head pain, this would appear to be an irrelevant detail.

When a medical professional interviews a new patient, it's similar to a detective interviewing a witness at a crime scene. And the patient (or witness, for patients are like witnesses to their own medical issues) may not realize what information will be most useful, will "solve the case." Lizzy might have dismissed or overlooked the fact that she began to suffer after yoga class because the connection didn't occur to her, or to any of the health professionals she'd seen to date, as significant. Largely this was due to the acceptance of current medical wisdom—that trigeminal neuralgia is caused by the blood vessel in the head. End of story. But Lizzy was telling me a different story.

My general view is that if a particular movement or incident triggered pain, then there's a good chance we can unravel whatever got tangled up and restore harmony in the body. But it was a big

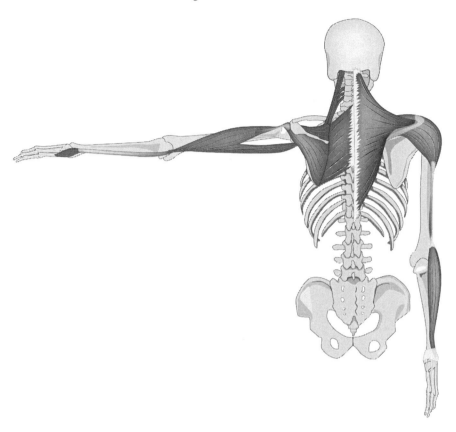

Muscles in the arm, shoulder blade and neck are connected via fascia creating a web of communication between distant tissues.

leap to suspect that I could apply this thinking to a problem deep in the skull. That was a connection I'd not yet considered, much less mastered.

There's a parable of a tugboat captain whose boat broke. He called a repairman who spent the next hour tapping valves and pipes, tugging on wires and pressing buttons as he evaluated the problem. Finally, in the end, he took out his hammer, tapped a small lever and the engine started up. He presented his bill to the tugboat captain: $1,000.

"But all you did was tap a lever!" the captain complained.

"Oh, it was $1 to tap the lever, $999 to know where to tap," replied the repairman.

11. *Pain Is a Sandcastle*

That's the value of understanding a system and how each component fits together. When you understand the system, interventions seem too simplistic—I hear that all the time. "I can't believe my back feels so much better just by unlocking my knees!" some would say. Or strengthening Al's gluteal muscles. Or taping Deb's shoulder.

That's me just tapping the right lever.

Anyone can learn to do what I do.

I needed to find Lizzy's lever and began by going after the biggest culprit, her shoulder blade. I moved it and massaged the deep muscle spasms that were locking it in an abnormal position. I read her face for signs of pain, but I thought nothing I could do would compare to the agony she experienced on a daily basis. Her pain tolerance had skyrocketed for the unfortunate reason of having suffered so much for so long. I then taped the shoulder blade into a better position.

After her first session with me, three new things happened with Lizzy. First, her pain decreased significantly and leveled off that day. Second, she slept through the night with no pain. Third, she forgot to take her pain meds for an hour and a half—she hadn't missed them for months.

The trigeminal nerve has a central portion called a subnucleus caudalis that extends all the way down through the brainstem and into the upper part of the neck around the second or third vertebra below the skull. I think of the nucleus like an egg yolk—it's the center of everything that happens in a cell. There's a portion of this nucleus that sends pain and temperature signals to the brain.

The shoulder blade has a muscle, the levator scapula, that attaches to the upper neck vertebrae at the same level as the trigeminal "egg yolk." I knew that Lizzy had a history of left-sided problems—shoulder dislocation and auto accidents left her with migraines and other symptoms. I'd had success fixing such things in the past by removing stress to the levator scapula. Maybe this would help release the nerve root fingers' hold on the trigeminal egg yolk?

It seemed to work. Simple, when you think about it.

As I mentioned, the trigeminal nerve has a unique architecture in that the nucleus that controls pain and temperature, subnucleus caudalis, extends down through the brainstem all the way to the upper cervical vertebral levels of C2 and C3. This nucleus also receives information from three other cranial nerves: facial (CN VII),

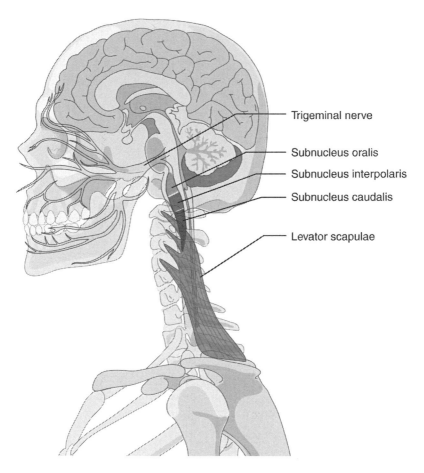

Trigeminal nerve

Subnucleus oralis

Subnucleus interpolaris

Subnucleus caudalis

Levator scapulae

The subnucleus caudalis of the trigeminal nerve extends down to vertebral levels C2 or C3 which allows it to be influenced by levator scapula inserting to those spinal levels.

glossopharyngeal (CN IX) and vagus (CN X). The vagus nerve has recently become a popular nerve to address due to its role in regulating internal organ functions. The facial cranial nerve helps control facial muscles but is also responsible for a large portion of taste receptors on our tongue. The glossopharyngeal cranial nerve also has a role in taste. Recall that Lizzy complained that her sense of taste had been altered.

So the trigeminal nerve is a big deal and communicates with

other cranial nerves too. I wasn't aware of this until long after my success with Lizzy.

When I first saw Lizzy, I vaguely remembered there was a trigeminal nerve. Cranial nerves are among the things we memorize in PT school and promptly forget afterward because we rarely deal with them—at least in orthopedics. So after meeting Lizzy, I gave myself a crash course in trigeminal nerve anatomy. The most important aspect of this, that the subnucleus caudalis extends down to C2 and C3, didn't come up in any of my searches. It was only after visiting the cadaver lab at nearby Regis University where I mobilized shoulder blades to understand exactly which tissues I was affecting during that maneuver that I was able to get an answer. Just before I was about to leave, the anatomy professor came in and I swooped down immediately, relating Lizzy's case.

"Why do you think I was able to help her by mobilizing her scapula?" I asked. "It must have something to do with the levator scapula,"

"Must be the subnucleus caudalis," he replied.

"What's that?" I asked, having never come across it.

"It extends down to C2 or C3."

I was terribly excited because my success with Lizzy was a few years before this conversation and I still couldn't get her out of my mind—I suppose I can be a bit obsessive about things.

I went back and searched "subnucleus caudalis" and pieced together the information you're reading today. I don't have this encyclopedic knowledge of the body in my head at all times. I remember the things that are meaningful.

The second idea I incorporated had to do with the points along her arms that triggered her symptoms. Nothing works in isolation in the body and one of the tissues that makes this a reality is fascia. Fascia is connective tissue that holds everything in place—muscles, blood vessels, nerve, viscera (our guts) and more. There are "highways" of fascia that run through our body. One runs from the hands to the head. This is why pressing anywhere on either arm elicited symptoms in her face—I was pressing her fascial web, delivering tension to the neck.

Think of that trigeminal egg yolk as the weakest and most irritated link in that web-chain. The fascia has a tendency to contract or become tight in the presence of injuries. Lizzy had quite a history of trauma from her car accidents and dislocated shoulder. So her fascia was already tighter than a drum before she headed into that fateful yoga class. The yoga simply added to her supersaturated condition, pushing it over the edge. Trigeminal neuralgia was the solid precipitate that fell from her concentrate.

In my simple way of looking at things, I figured that if this highway can irritate the trigeminal nerve, then it could also calm it down. So part of our treatment was gently massaging the main points along this fascial canal to reduce the tension in the web. It seemed to have worked.

During our third session, while I was working on her shoulder, she turned to me. "It's like when you have a sandcastle and pour water on it and see it melt away. That's what I feel like when you're working with me—my pain is melting away."

I loved that analogy. It meant that my approach was helping. I felt I was indirectly reaching up into her brain, visualizing the connections between her shoulder blade and the trigeminal nerve branches infiltrating her face.

Over the next few weeks, I watched a woman I had never met emerge from under her dark cloud of pain and misery. I wish I could say she was miraculously better in three visits, but to be honest, we had a lot of work to do because of her extensive history of car accidents and the shoulder dislocation, none of which had been addressed adequately.

What I noticed, though, was that she smiled more and lost that metaphorical heaviness she'd had been carrying on her shoulders. The face mask was no longer needed. She was sleeping better too. When we sleep, we heal—our mind clears, and we see the world a little differently.

Further into our work together, Lizzy began photographing again and going out with her friends. She slowly, steadily reclaimed her life. She had a new future ahead of her now, one that she thought she'd never see again, like a lost loved one taken for granted until they were gone. Except this time, she could have them back.

After a few more treatments, we'd eliminated almost all of her pain, including the fishhook in the face feeling, the broken glass in her nose, the sensitivity to light and sound. There was no more dizziness or nausea. She had weaned off her pain medications and she was sleeping much better.

She was about 85 percent better when she learned that her insurance wouldn't pay for any more sessions. I got on the phone to argue her case, but nothing on my part could convince them otherwise. It was a bureaucratic decision: the policy was that X number of sessions were covered and that was it, regardless of the situation. Before she stopped coming in, I taught her how to continue on her own so that she could achieve full recovery. I still think of her often, hoping she's out there laughing, enjoying the mountains and taking beautiful pictures.

≈ 12 ≋

Fear Can Be a Pain
in the Neck

I still have the silver dollar. On one side of it, my father inscribed the word FEAR. On the other side? FREEDOM. He pressed it into my hand when, long ago in my early 20s, I set off to travel the world.

"On the other side of fear is freedom," he would say. By this he meant that, if you face your fears, you can free yourself from them. Dad's silver coin reminded me to take time to think about my fears when deciding whether or not to move forward. Fear can inhibit but it can also empower. And fear is healthy. It makes you think before you act.

Well, now my daughter has my silver dollar. I gave it to her one night when she was having a bad dream and couldn't fall back asleep. I told her this story and said that her dreams were just in her head. Understand that they're only in your imagination and you're free of them. I wish I'd been told this about my own self-doubt. I still wrestle it, even though an objective observer would say that I've proven myself and I should be well past it. She clasped the silver dollar in her small hand and quickly fell asleep.

For my son's 16th birthday, my daughter and I bought him an identical silver dollar. She chose the coin and we took it to the engraver together. My son wants to see the world and I thought this would be a good companion for him, as it's been for me and my daughter.

I explored the world solo, with no companion save my journal and the occasional traveler whose path ran parallel to mine for a spell. Because I wandered alone, I became acutely aware of my thoughts and moods. Often I found myself worrying about something but I wasn't sure exactly what or why. I would then sit down with my journal and write about it. This would expose underlying fears that had snuck up on me. My journal allowed me to see them. It was like a lantern in the darkness. Seeing them helped me address them.

I was a budget traveler, and this was a time before the Internet or mobile phones. The transportation I took and the places I stayed were rarely in the safest parts of town. I was often squeezed into the humanity of the places I visited: Australia (where I celebrated my 23rd birthday), New Zealand, Japan (my 24th birthday), South Korea, China (25th birthday), Hong Kong, Indonesia, Thailand, Nepal, India, Egypt, Kenya (26th birthday), Uganda, Zaire, Burundi, Rwanda, Tanzania, Malawi. The smells, sounds, foods and livestock were constant sources of entertainment and wonder to me.

My fears were usually of things out of my control. Would there be a place for me to sleep? How would I get from the bus or train station to a hostel? If I was arriving in the evening, were there criminals waiting to relieve me of my money and passport? Could I trust the smiling taxi driver who offered to take me where I wanted to go?

These fears, if left unaddressed, would build to a raging whitewater of worry that washed through my mind and body. A sense of unease or a nagging feeling of dread would hang over me. I learned to identify them as soon as they appeared on my radar and to see them for what they were: circumstances I could be aware of but not control. The best I could do was to plan for whatever awaited me.

Because I couldn't understand what most people were saying, I learned to read their faces, gestures and body language. I developed a sense of intuition about people as a result. This helped me read situations, anything from buying food in a marketplace to crossing a border. I learned to trust in my ability to handle whatever was presented to me. As my confidence grew, my gnawing worries abated.

My silver coin, nestled in my money belt close against my skin, reminded me to face my fears. With my newly honed sense of intuition and awareness, I grew more comfortable with the unknown. Later, this would help me recognize fear and anxiety in others.

Solving the Pain Puzzle

Beverley drove an hour and a half to see me. I always feel more pressure when someone visits my clinic from far away. These people took the time to seek me out and have high expectations of my ability to heal them. I felt like I was being tested, like in PT school when an instructor would pull me to the front of the class to have me demonstrate an evaluation technique. I was on the spot. I thought I needed to pack in as much as possible for Beverley and wow her a little, so as not to disappoint.

Beverley had suffered from chronic migraines, neck pain and numbness in both hands for several years and was desperate for help. She was in her mid–20s and in excellent condition. She had been in a couple of car accidents in the past two years, each worsening her symptoms to the point where she was having a hard time functioning at school and work. She rarely smiled and had furrowed eyebrows. I imagined that these were a result of her war with pain. This was not the face of a carefree twenty-something.

While I was evaluating her, I noticed that she couldn't relax enough to allow her arms and hands to be floppy. I could see her wincing even with my light touch as I probed different muscles in her arms, shoulders and neck.

I performed all my usual tests, found the usual suspects that would contribute to her pain and we began working to untangle them. After a few sessions together, we saw little improvement. I felt terrible because she was driving so far to see me. But even more, I grew suspicious that something else was going on. This is one of the benefits of my approach; when I don't see a rapid change in pain, I can quickly move on to another potential source of it. Because my evaluation is comprehensive, I have a good idea of all the potential issues by the end of my exam.

"Beverley, I just want to look at something in your stomach," I said.

"Sure," she replied.

I asked her to lie down on her back while I slowly pressed down on her stomach until I reached what I thought was a deep muscle that lies along both sides of the spine, called the psoas.

To do this, I had to push through several other tissues, like the stomach muscles and digestive organs. At first blush, this might sound very aggressive and painful, but I can do it quite gently.

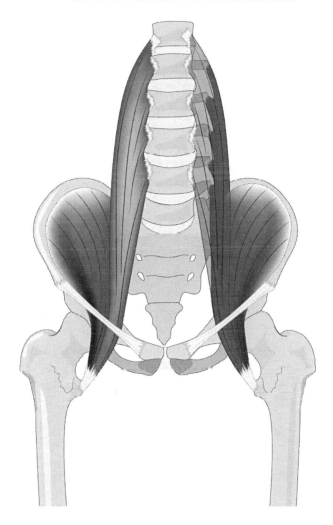

The psoas muscle lies deep to the viscera and connects the vertebrae of the lumbar spine to the hip bone. There are fascial connections traveling to the neck and head as well.

The key is to help the patient relax their stomach muscles. If they are tense, which many people are when I first touch them here, then I won't be successful. Beverley was no different.

"Okay, try to relax your stomach," I said. "I won't press hard here and, if you want me to stop, I will. I just need to check some muscles here that are a little deep."

She nodded and closed her eyes to help focus on relaxing her stomach. I slowly increased my pressure as she allowed me to go deeper. I watched her face to make sure she wasn't in pain.

I've learned over the years to pause just before I reach the psoas muscles. This is often a sensitive area for people even without chronic pain. As I get closer to my goal, patients tend to subconsciously contract their stomach muscles again. Pausing gives them a moment to relax and trust me and my presence there. As I paused with Beverley, I felt her mounting tension subside. This silent sign of trust allowed me to go just a little further toward my target.

I allowed my fingers to lightly brush the psoas muscles I was seeking. I looked for tissue that was a little too hard. I subtly allowed the ends of my fingertips to bend back, so I could use the softer pads of my fingers, rather than the bony tips, which can be painful. There are more nerve endings in my finger pads than the tips, which allowed me to sense the tissues better.

As I suspected, Beverley's psoas muscles harbored small knots of tissue. When I encountered one, I pressed slightly more firmly and waited for her response. She cringed and I noticed what seemed to be a fleeting look of nervousness on her face. I cautiously explored this muscle on both sides of her spine, feeling for knots, occasionally glancing at her face.

"I feel that up in my neck," she said. Her voice was just a half-pitch higher than usual. The words were slightly rushed, the eyebrows raised just a smidge.

My radar picked up something. I'd seen this before—in myself and other patients. Fear? Worry? Or was this more?

⇒⇐ ⇒⇐ ⇒⇐

The Diagnostic and Statistical Manual of Mental Disorders (*DSM*) is a guide for health care workers to diagnose mental health disorders. It is periodically updated and, as I write, the *DSM* is in its fifth incarnation—*DSM-5.*

The *DSM-5* states that generalized anxiety disorder is characterized by "excessive anxiety and worry (apprehensive expectation), occurring more days than not for at least 6 months, about a number of events or activities (such as work or school performance)." Furthermore, "the person finds it difficult to control the worry."

12. *Fear Can Be a Pain in the Neck*

I had a lot of my own experiences of fear and worry, first while traveling and then when having a family of my own, as well as my perceived failures as a PT and my trepidation about writing and publishing my books, including this one.

Fear and worry abound, fed by the constant drone of news outlets and social media reporting new tragedies springing up apparently out of our control. If left unchecked, these fears and worries would induce anxiety even in people who are not prone to it. One of my patients described her anxiety as a physical expression of fear—something she could feel throughout her body.

I decided to gently query Beverley.

"Do you suffer from anxiety?" I asked.

Her eyes widened. "How did you know that?"

I explained that it was a lot of little things: her posture, the tension and tone of her muscles, her lack of progress and, finally, the irritation of her psoas muscles, together with her facial and voice cues.

She shared that she'd been dealing with anxiety for years.

The psoas muscles begin in the front of the lower back, deep to our guts, and insert into the tops of the thigh bones. They have connections to all five vertebra of the lower back and the discs between them. But why would I look to the psoas muscles for clues to Beverley's pain in her neck?

When we are born, we have reflexes hardwired into our brains and bodies that help us negotiate the world and develop as babies. One of these is the Landau Reflex that triggers our back muscles to contract, arching the back and lifting our heads. When we begin to move and crawl, we tap into this reflex so we can see where we're going.

It also comes into play when we need to be alert. Think of walking through a forest and hearing a loud snap of a branch near you. You freeze with your head up, back straight and eyes wide open, suddenly alert to every noise around you. That deep Landau Reflex is partially responsible for this unconscious response to help you assess a situation and be ready to respond to potential danger.

Another is a withdrawal reflex that, when our foot touches something unexpected or painful, triggers one side of our body to contract its muscles to pull that foot away from the stimulus. This happens in the blink of an eye. Imagine stepping, barefoot, onto a shard of glass. This hidden reflex helps you pull that foot away pronto, to keep you safe from further damage. This recruits waist and leg muscles to keep you safe.

Yet another is a startle reflex, in response to a falling sensation or loud sounds. This causes us to contract our arms and legs to protect our body. You can see this at work in pictures of people who are frightened. Their shoulders shrug up and they hunch over slightly to protect their vital organs and head. This pattern recruits many of the muscles in the front of our trunk, like the chest, abdominals and arm.

While these reflexes disappear at varying ages, the hardwiring remains. The reflex responses are overridden by our higher cerebral functions which allow us to deal with other concerns during the day. After all, we can't go through life reflexively responding to every event or sound.

I see the psoas muscles as part of the startle reflex pattern of contraction. They activate in response to fear stimuli, among other things. They are implicated in back pain, but I've found that they come into play with digestive issues, like gluten intolerance or Crohn's disease, and psychological issues, like anxiety, depression or trauma. These chronic issues seem to cause the psoas muscles to remain contracted and thus create the knots I was finding in Beverley.

This general description of the reflex patterns is part of the Hanna Somatics approach to solving pain. I tend to agree with it. Looking at the startle reflex pattern of contraction, to me the psoas seems to be an element of this. Interestingly, just as Dr. Shirley Sahrmann and Dr. Thomas Hanna describe three very similar patterns of dysfunction behind back pain, Thomas Meyers, a fascia expert, also identifies "super highways" of fascia running through the body that are virtually identical to Hanna and Sahrmann's description in his book *Anatomy Trains*.

There is no muscular attachment from the psoas muscle up to Beverley's neck that would account for her pain there. You might be wondering, then, why am I dragging you through Beverley's psoas muscles if there's no connection to her neck? For that, you need to understand just one more player in this mystery—fascia.

Fascia is tissue that holds everything together in our body like a web. Sometimes these strands are gossamer threads while others are broad, tough swaths of tissue, like bolts of fabric. These larger fascial tracts allow different areas and structures of the body to communicate with and influence one another. The brain is the spider constantly monitoring this web, unconsciously making small adjustments here and there.

The referral of pain from Beverley's psoas muscles to her neck told me that her anxiety issues, which were potentially causing her psoas muscles to contract, may be contributing to her neck pain, migraines and ultimately the numbness in her hands via these fascial pathways.

What this meant for Beverley was that we needed to calm her nervous system while also fixing the mechanical causes of her neck pain. Calming the nervous system helps reduce the effects of anxiety on the body by calming the muscles too.

While we hear about the mind/body connection almost daily, it's entirely another thing to manipulate that connection to achieve a physical outcome. Luckily, years ago, I learned a nifty technique that allows me to do just this.

Often, when working with the nervous system in this way, I remember when my son, Boone, was born. He was placed on a table, screaming, while the nurse tended to him. She monitored his heart rate while I gently placed my hand on his little head.

"He knows you," she said, "his heart rate went down when you touched his head."

We have billions of nerve endings that lie between one and six millimeters deep in our skin. These nerves are one way that our brain monitors the world around us. This means that we all are at least two millimeters away from directly impacting each other's brains through touch. That's less than 1/10th of an inch—a few sheets of paper. We're closer to making deep connections with each other than we might realize.

What this meant for Beverley and me was that, because our nerve endings were basically touching each other, she could read my nervous system just as I was trying to affect hers. I needed to remain calm to help her relax. I slowed my breathing, quietly exhaling longer than I inhaled. This stimulated a portion of my nervous system that promotes relaxation. I was also aware that Beverley would, on some level, listen to my breathing and pick up on those nonverbal cues subconsciously. I felt my heart rate slow, and my gaze soften, to take all of her in, scanning for signs of relaxation.

Having this time to be present with a patient is increasingly rare in medicine. Just ask any doctor, if you can slow them down enough, that is. The economics of medicine, particularly in the United States, drive doctors to reduce one-on-one patient time to just a few minutes. This often makes it difficult to connect meaningfully with patients. I'm always surprised that physicians do as well as they do, with the little time they have.

As a physical therapist, though, I have the luxury of establishing a relationship, taking in the non-verbal cues and interpreting them, tracing a pattern of problems to their source and generally getting to know my patients on a deeper level. This allowed me to make quicker connections with Beverley's problems. Being slower, more deliberate, actually sped things up in terms of identifying the problem.

The key to this technique was to stimulate the nerve endings in her skin. The funny thing about the nerves in our skin is that each responds to a different kind of stimulus. Some respond to light stroking, while their neighbors remain unaffected. But those same neighbors might respond to scratching or tapping instead, allowing the stroking nerves to remain calm and rested.

For this technique to work, there were five different types of nerves I was interested in stimulating: light stroking, tapping, vibration, deep pressure and light scratching. I devoted a few minutes to each for her arms and legs. This took about 30 minutes. I think of it as a long, slow reset of her nervous system.

While working with her, I watched and listened to her body. The tone of her muscles, the gurgle of her stomach, the cadence of her breath and the ease of her joint motions all suggested her parasympathetic nervous system, her rest-and-digest system, was coming online. This is what I hoped for.

When I finished, she groggily opened her eyes. "Oh my gosh," she yawned, "I can't remember when I've been so relaxed." Her speech was slower, she didn't move her body, and her voice dropped a couple of notes lower—more signs that she was calmer.

In spite of an hour-and-a-half drive back home that evening, she had no migraines or neck pain. Nor the next day. This hadn't happened in the previous two years. We both knew what this meant: her pain was caused, in a large part, by her anxiety, which was locking down her body in a particular pattern that triggered neck pain and headaches. The pathway seemed to be that the anxiety activated her psoas muscles along both sides of her lower spine, which then referred pain up to her neck and head via fascial connections.

The treatment I gave her helped release its hold temporarily— enough to see how much it contributed to her pain, which was a lot. Together we formed a plan for her to see a psychologist in parallel to my work on the mechanical problems.

Three months later, I was happily surprised to see Beverley on my schedule. She practically bounced into my clinic. No furrowed brow to be seen.

"I'm completely better!" she said. "I haven't had a headache in over a month! I just wanted you to check out my physical problems." She was beaming.

"That's great, Beverley! How did you do it?" I asked.

"I've been seeing a counselor who's been helping me while I did the PT exercises you gave me on my own. My anxiety is so much better. I feel like a new person. And no pain at all!"

"I'm so happy for you!"

Beverley chose to face her fears, worries and anxiety, and now she is free of them—along with her pain. I was not privy to her personal struggles, but I know that this was no simple task. Most of us would much rather work with a physical problem than a mental one. But, in Beverley's case, she had a chance to see exactly how much her psychological issues were breaking down her body.

The choice was clear.

She faced her fear and found her freedom.

⇛ 13 ⇚

Falling in the Same
River Twice

"No man ever steps in the same river twice, for it's not the same river and he's not the same man." Greek philosopher Heraclitus knew what he was talking about. But instead of stepping into the river, I fell in.

I prided myself on helping people quickly get out of pain and back to their lives. Andrea blew my average out of the water, though. And for one of the simplest problems I tend to see at the clinic—knee pain.

Andrea was a vibrant young woman in her late 20s, already with a young family. She lit up a room when entering and had a loud, infectious laugh. I could hear her from the next room as she waited, joking with my receptionist.

She came to see me for chronic knee pain which began a few years earlier. She had already had several knee surgeries. This was a little surprising for someone so young and who didn't play competitive sports. My radar was up a little—something different was happening here.

During my evaluation I found several problems common to knees such as hypermobility (ligaments and joints that are too loose), her knees locked backward when she walked or stood, and butt muscle weakness. We worked through these issues, but her pain remained the same. Even my miracle muscle massage to the popliteus behind the knee didn't work. Another red flag.

I then began my back-up plan. I looked further away from the knee into the foot and hip. I taped her flat feet to lift her arches. I attacked her hip weakness. I mobilized her hip joints to put them in a better position. No luck. Louder alarms went off in my head now.

13. *Falling in the Same River Twice*

On our seventh visit I tried some deep tissue massage to her legs. About 10 minutes into our session, I noticed a twitch in one of her arms. At the same time her eyes blinked hard as if a loud explosion had just occurred.

"I'm sorry, did I hurt you?" I asked.

"No, why?" she said.

"Oh, just that twitch in your arm and you blinked hard. I thought I hit a tender spot," I replied.

"I wasn't aware of any twitch," she said.

My alarm went off again. I hadn't picked up any signs of excessive muscle tension in her body during our evaluation but that could be because she was a hypermobile person. These people tend to be too loose rather than stiff so it's harder to pick up tension-related changes in muscle tone.

Hypermobility is a term I use for people whose joints move just a little too much. Joints are limited not only by their bony architecture but also by muscles and ligaments. Muscles contract to control joints but ligaments don't. They connect bone to bone and are the primary guides of our joint movements.

Think of Sallie's left foot that had collapsed. Her bag of potatoes was too loose. Hypermobile people have looser bags than the rest of us. We need some tension in our ligaments to hold the bones in place properly so our muscles can move them ideally. Ligaments in this way assist muscles so they don't become too strained and overworked. I think of ligaments as primary controllers of joints. Muscles are secondary controllers.

We tend to do more of the things we're good at. Hypermobile people gravitate to disciplines like dance, yoga, Pilates, gymnastics, and swimming. They believe stretching is the way to solve pain like a weightlifter thinks strengthening is the best way to fix a problem.

There are drawbacks to hypermobility, though. Muscles develop painful knots from overexertion of picking up the slack (so to speak) for ligaments that aren't helping them. These muscles are usually too long themselves. Joint surfaces become irritated because the ligaments and muscles aren't controlling them nicely and absorbing shock. That's why hypermobile people have their share of aches and pains too.

The contortionists you see performing for crowds at an outdoor mall, *America's Got Talent*, or Cirque du Soleil are extremely hyper-mobile people. I can't watch their performances without thinking about the pain they must be in. So if you find yourself competing to get that foot behind your head in yoga like your instructor, think again. It may not be the best thing for you, or them.

"I know this is a little weird, but have you had some kind of emotional trauma in your life?" I queried.

"Well, yes, some," she said, caught a little off guard. Her smile vanished.

I finished our visit with the deep tissue massage. I didn't expect her knee pain to change when she came in for her next session and I was right.

"Today, we're going to do something a little different, Andrea," I said. "I'm going to try to calm down your nervous system to see if that helps your pain. Is that okay with you?" I asked.

"Yeah, sure," she said, "but why did you ask about emotional trauma before?" She looked worried.

"Because you might be holding on to something that is causing tension in your knees. Today I just want to see if there's anything to that theory," I replied.

Pain from trauma can be expressed in a particular muscle or area of the body, similar to change to Beverley. I remember working out deep knots in a man's inner thigh muscles to resolve his hip pain. The tension and knots kept returning, though.

"Why are you holding so much tension here, Barry?" I said, half to myself.

"Do you mean because my mom abandoned us when I was five years old?" he said. Tears then gushed. "I don't know why I just said that," he confessed. "I haven't told anyone about that. Could that have something to do with it?"

"That very well could be the reason," I said gently after he calmed down. His inner thigh tension was much reduced after that session.

I applied my technique for calming Andrea's sympathetic nervous system (her fight or flight nervous system). It was the same process I used with Beverley earlier.

I began with her right arm then moved to her left leg. Both shoulders suddenly jerked forward off the table and back again. It was as if an electric shock just ripped through her body. It startled us both.

"What was that?!" she asked, rattled.

"I think you just let go of some of that trauma I was wondering about," I said. "When you relax more deeply, old patterns of trauma surface which have been held in your body and are released in the form of a large twitch."

"What do you mean?" she said, sounding anxious.

I explained to her there is a theory that when we experience trauma, our body will move into a freeze response whereby we are rendered incapable of moving. This happens especially in times when we feel we can't escape the event.

This can be seen in the animal kingdom when prey are caught. Typing in *trauma release animals* on YouTube will show some videos about this. They go into a deep trance-like state presumably to avoid the horror of being killed and eaten. Their sympathetic nervous system energy is overruled by a deeper freeze response from an older part of the brain. Dr. Peter Levine writes extensively about this in his amazing book *In an Unspoken Voice*.

Sometimes if the predator is distracted, has to fight off other predators for the kill, or walks away due to lack of interest, the prey snaps out of their trance and is able to get up and run away. Often the prey will later shake or tremble in parts of its body, releasing stored sympathetic nervous system energy.

This happens in humans too. The twitch is the body's way of releasing that deeper stored energy from trauma they haven't been able to release before. I often wonder if this is what happens with me, just as I'm falling asleep, when my arm or leg twitches, waking me up. Unfortunately, we're not always aware of the presence of this energy because our higher-level cognitive brain functions override that release.

"If you'd like to stop here, we can," I said. I was treading on shaky territory because I knew Andrea hadn't been seeing a therapist or counselor. I didn't know anything about the trauma she faced and wasn't equipped to handle that type of problem. She agreed to stop, but the next session she asked to do it again.

"I'm just curious if it was a one-time thing," she said. I was too.

I began the treatment again, and when I reached the left leg, she had a big twitch in her left arm.

"Keep going," she said, a little worried. "I want to see if it happens again."

I continued my treatment, and when I got to her left arm, it happened again. And then her right leg as well. She looked a little panicked.

"I don't understand. Why is this happening?" she asked, nearly sobbing.

"I think you've got some deeper trauma locked in your body. This might be why you're having chronic knee pain. Your body is experiencing tension from this trauma and your knees are the weakest links," I said.

"I don't like it," she said. After a few more moments, she added, "But I think you might be right."

"If I'm right, then you need to see a counselor if you want me to continue. You need a professional to help you deal with this. This isn't my specialty," I said.

Andrea found a therapist and they began their work while also continuing with me. One of my goals as a PT is to rapidly reduce pain and restore function. But this would take time. I had to adjust my expectations—I was in for the long term with Andrea.

We met once a week. Andrea would jerk in spasms while we released her tension. I was often uncomfortable being there with her, I'm ashamed to say. I focused on her experience, though. She needed this to happen. We were in the trenches facing it together.

Our time together helped me see the privilege of my job. To be deeply connected with another person is not common in most professions. That connection is possible through their willingness to be vulnerable.

Andrea was vulnerable with me in ways that perhaps she wasn't even with her family. This is, in my opinion, one of the gifts of being human, this ability to connect on many levels with another, in many different ways.

Eventually Andrea became less emotional about the spasms and started looking at them more objectively. We commented about the degree and timing of them as if they were things separate from her. Objectifying them helped calm her and conquer her fear.

At the end of the day, I returned home silent and tired, ate dinner and went to bed. Throughout our time together, I wondered if we were doing the right thing. This was uncharted territory for me. The human mind and body are vastly interconnected, and those connections are complex. I had to be comfortable not knowing where this was heading.

Almost a year had passed when we noticed her spasms began to occur later into the treatment. Eventually they became minor tremors. Finally, there were no tremors at all. Whether I had anything to do with it or not, I still don't know.

"I'm so excited about this!" said Andrea one day. "They're changing!"

On her own, Andrea worked on her strengthening and stretching exercises throughout our sessions together.

At the end of the year, she had virtually no knee pain. She was also a different person. The perky, vivacious young woman with a quick, loud laugh was replaced with a more self-assured individual. She seemed calmer, for lack of a better description. Content.

How did soothing her nervous system help with her emotional trauma? The short answer is I don't know. What I do know is that her pain seemed to be an expression of her trauma—the canary in her coal mine. Calming her nervous system had the effect of calming her mind by releasing the physical expression of that trauma. And vice versa.

I won't discount the fact that we developed a bond while working together that went deeper than most I have with my patients. I was one of the few people who saw her at her most vulnerable. Her loud, vivacious personality hung outside the door at each visit. As time went on, she seemed content to leave it there.

She taught me that being there for someone can be enough. I don't always have to do something. I now sit quietly when occasionally patients shed tears at my table, rather than rush to console them. They can let it out and I can be silent. They are quiet moments where we are fully human together.

I think about Andrea often and wonder how she's doing. I don't dare check in on her as I feel I might be a reminder of a painful time in her life that she'd rather put behind her. I hope she might see our time together, though, as a period where she shed her past and emerged a more aware person in control of her life.

⇒ 14 ⇐

The Three Pillars of Pain (and How to Topple Them)

My three-year-old son ran across the playground, screaming with joy. I watched his chubby little legs occasionally misstep, almost tripping him up. Then he fell with what looked to be extraordinary force, hitting the ground hard. "How could that little body generate so much impact?" I marveled to myself. He looked up at my wife and me. She snapped into action.

"Boone, are you okay?! Oh my, are you hurt?" she yelled while running to him, her voice shrill.

His eyes then filled with tears, and he started crying. Make that screaming.

At this, I stood up and walked toward him slowly. My wife had him in her arms.

"Oh my goodness, what a fall. I bet that hurt! Let me look at you," she said to him while holding his sobbing body close to hers. "Oh my gosh, look at those scrapes. My poor boy."

"Let's take a look, Boone," I said when I got there. I looked at the scrapes on his forehead, elbow and knees. He was covered with dirt and his nose was running from crying.

"Wow, that was your best fall yet! Nice job, Boone!" I laughed. "Let's check you out. Man, I wish I had scrapes like that. You must be so proud of yourself. Can you move your arms and legs? Great! Ready to go again?"

And with that, he was up and running.

It took me a little while to help my wife change her reaction to our kids' accidents. I saw that our kids started crying only after checking on us parents to see how we reacted. If we waved them on, then they'd just get up and hop back to it. If we made a big deal of it, they reveled in, or fed off, our concern and started crying, welcoming the comfort we offered. It was up to us—they were fine.

Slowly but surely, my wife's reaction shifted from fear and worry to calm appraisal. First assess to see if any real damage was done. Give kids a chance to get up on their own. Hold them calmly, if that's what they need, and praise them for whatever they were doing when they fell. Let them know you love them. Then let them go.

To her credit, and against her instincts, my wife eventually mastered the idea. I think our kids were the better for it.

Later, when our kids had an accident, they would turn to us and be met with a "Nice job!" or "Whoa, that was a big one!" or "Wow, that was cool!" They would then get up and continue playing, happy that nothing was really wrong.

Many years later, my cousin, David, and I took my two kids canoeing and camping in Quetico National Park in Canada. It's a remote park with no amenities and great expanses of lakes and rivers.

Edie was 11 and Boone was 13. David and I paddled fiercely for about six hours our first day. We finally found a place to camp on an island after nearly capsizing from a sudden squall. Our campsite was a sloping slab of granite with small trees and grass growing out of it.

Freezing rain and wind pelted us for the two nights we camped. During the day it was windy. Our sleeping bags were drenched after the first night and remained cold and damp the entire trip. The wind and waves were so strong that we couldn't even get our canoe on the lake to fish the next day. Instead, I blazed a trail on our small island to get to the other side. I caught one walleye and we fried it up for dinner.

The second night, we listened to the cold, steady rain pelt our tent. Thunder and lightning rolled through all night long. A large branch poked into my back from below. I frequently awoke to cracks of thunder and watched my breath. My kids slowly slid toward the bottom of the slope on which the tent was pitched, inching down to the lower corner of our tent, where the water collected.

The next morning, Boone sat up in his sleeping bag. Water dripped from his zipper. That was the morning we were due to break camp to return home. My cousin and I cut our tarp into ponchos for the kids to keep them as dry and warm as possible for the journey home. Then we paddled through a freezing drizzle. Even covered, the kids shivered the whole way back. I could barely feel my hands. My cousin could hardly stand up once we hit shore.

That wasn't all. Mosquitos swarmed us after we landed. We had about a quarter-mile portage with our gear and boat uphill to get to the pick-up location. A small stream formed along the path, making the portage hazardous. Once all the gear was up from the lake, a van eventually arrived. We loaded our gear, and hungry, frozen and exhausted, we returned to our cabin in northern Minnesota four hours later. The cabin is owned by my Uncle Dave. I've taken the kids there for years, since they were small, to go fishing, eat s'mores and live on Kitchi Lake for about a week at a time. Growing up in urban Denver, they never had a chance to experience wilderness like that. It's one thing I felt I did right as a dad, taking them there every year. My cousin David's cabin was just 50 yards from mine and the kids would run between the two. It was here that they shot their first bow and arrow, BB gun and shotgun, caught their first fish, ate their first s'more, swam in their first lake, caught their first snake, got bitten by their first mosquito. We always went up on Father's Day each year and I was in heaven traveling with them, knowing they were going to have a wonderful time.

The fallout from the Quetico trip was divided. My son couldn't wait to go back. My daughter never would. In fact, that was the last time she joined us in Minnesota. Both had the same experience but internalized it differently.

There is an emotional component to pain. That aspect can be learned. Just like when my kids were small and looked to us for cues as to how to react to their accidents. If we screamed and acted panicky, they became afraid and cried, no doubt feeling their injury more.

But reactions are also hardwired in our brains, like my daughter refusing to return to Minnesota and my son chomping at the bit every year. Both had the same experience of childhood, the same parents, but they processed it differently. Pain becomes a stew comprised of learned reactions, hardwiring in our DNA, and physical problems. As a therapist, sometimes I need to tease these out to understand what's at the bottom of an issue.

I have had a surprising number of patients with chronic pain who have been resistant to the physical and psychological approaches I've tried with them. Surprising to others, who assume that anyone would be delighted to have pain alleviated. Not surprising to me. As a medical practitioner, I treat the human condition but live daily in the cloudy echo chamber of the human mind, seeing how it can powerfully affect the body, for good and for ill. Our minds are comprised of what we're born with mixed with what we experience, are taught and absorb as fact and truth.

There is one last ingredient to consider: things we ingest. Not metaphorically, like ideas, but literally. By this I mean the foods we eat and the air we breathe.

People have food allergies or sensitivities. Consuming these foods can cause the body to become inflamed, contributing to pain. I once had a client with chronic pain who discovered she was allergic to her favorite food which she ate all the time—watermelon. She cut this food out of her diet and her pain reduced by approximately 25 percent.

When patients stump me, I often suspect gluten intolerance as a possible source of irritation. Gluten is found in breads and pastas and can cause inflammation in those who are sensitive to it. It's the most obvious and easiest ingredient to eliminate from a diet. Anything beyond this I refer to a doctor or dietician. Diet and allergies aren't my specialty. But I see how often they affect physical therapy issues.

This category also includes things we breathe in, such as pollen and mold. Both can severely affect our bodies, creating an inflammatory condition. There are many books addressing these problems. It is more pervasive than you might think.

⇒⊂ ⇒⊂ ⇒⊂

Michelle was a longtime client of mine from my days working at a health club in downtown Denver. Although she didn't participate in sports, she was incredibly athletic and would quickly master any challenge I put to her. During our off days, she would spend hours working out in a home gym she'd built in her basement, outfitted with all the best equipment. Pound for pound, she was stronger and leaner than anyone at the club, which was filled with all sorts of elite athletes. She was simply amazing.

However, long ago, she developed some strange symptoms we

couldn't figure out. She would sometimes experience numbness and shaking of the left side of her body, which would pass after an hour or two. She would also complain of strange head pain and fatigue that might last a few days and then disappear. Additionally, her heart would sometimes race, even while she rested, and she sometimes had difficulty breathing.

Over the years we tried all sorts of ideas to help isolate the precipitating factors for these complaints. There was no discernible musculoskeletal cause or trigger, so we focused on her diet.

Michelle was also seeing a dietician and her food intake was pristine. No extra calories or processed foods. She was disciplined and would comply with whatever was recommended, 100 percent. This helped us quickly eliminate sources of triggers. The problem was that we ran out of ideas.

Michelle thought to visit a naturopathic doctor, an ND. NDs typically attend a four-year graduate program and are educated in basic sciences, like medical doctors. Their education also focuses on environmental and holistic medical intervention.

This doctor discovered that Michelle had, at one time, Lyme disease. Named after a small town in Connecticut where it was first discovered, Lyme disease is transmitted by a tick and can have far-reaching chronic effects on the body, including fatigue, headaches, muscle aches and more. I had heard of Lyme disease and knew it caused chronic musculoskeletal pain, but that was about the extent of it. To us, this likely explained Michelle's symptoms.

She received treatment and improved somewhat but never quite as much as we'd hoped. She decided to have further testing and her doctor found that she had traces of mold in her body. Mold spores are quite small and can be inhaled. At the time, I had no idea that mold could even be a factor in people's health. My focus was the musculoskeletal system and sometimes the mind-body connection. Mold was a completely new field for me.

Michelle's mold source was a mystery to us both; she lived in a very dry climate and her house was a relatively new build. Her workplace was also recently renovated, and no mold had been reported during the overhaul. She was a great cook and used only the freshest ingredients, so we didn't feel mold was coming into her body through her diet.

This mystery went on for years, as she continued to go to her ND for treatment. Then she and her husband decided to renovate their home. She wanted a new bedroom and bathroom, which took months to complete. During that renovation, she decided to change the flooring in her basement. When a worker pulled up a tile, it was completely black on the undersurface. Michelle literally screamed at the sight. She was mortified. They pulled up more tiles and found that her workout area was infested with black mold. Tracing it to the source, they discovered a gutter connection that had come loose and allowed water to stream down the side of the house. Over the years, it had migrated to the inside through small cracks in the mortar, above the dirt line, and traveled unseen behind the drywall, ending up in the basement.

Michelle wasted no time in tracing that leak, fixing it, and mitigating the mold. Within a few weeks, her symptoms abated and are overall about 90 percent improved, often 100 percent, she reports, unless her system becomes stressed by other factors.

To this day, Michelle's body is like a canary in a coal mine when it comes to mold. She has honed her awareness around this stressor. Recently, she went on vacation and walked into her hotel room. She instantly felt her sinuses begin to act up—there was mold in the room. She requested a new room in a different part of the hotel, one that was a newer construction, and had no symptoms at all.

≥⊏ ≥⊏ ≥⊏

Case studies like Michelle's helped me build up my overall Three Pillars of Pain theory. Think of pain as a line. Above that line, we experience pain. Below it, we do not. We want to stay below it. The line is our critical threshold.

There are three primary columns of issues pushing us up to this critical threshold of pain:

1. Physical problems like broken bones, muscle strains or the functional problems I've talked about causing strain to tissues, such as what happened to Al, Sallie and Jeni.
2. Psychological or emotional issues, like those of Beverley and Andrea.
3. Things we ingest like allergens, mold or gluten, as in Michelle's case.

Sometimes we reach our critical threshold from 100 percent of physical problems. Sometimes it's 40 percent emotional or psychological and 60 percent physical. And others its 50 percent things we ingest and 20 percent emotional or psychological and 30 percent physical. Everyone is different, each case a new combination of the Three Pillars.

There are myriad health and wellness books on the market. There are heal-your-back-pain books, like mine, anti-inflammatory diet books, and books that tout that all pain is from an emotional source. All of them are written by people who've had success using their approaches. All help some people and not others.

The Three Pillars of Pain explain why this is the case, why no one in medicine has a 100 percent success rate. There are just too many factors. Each patient brings their own recipe of genetics, history, psychology and physiology. Each medical practitioner brings their own recipe of training, experience, beliefs, successes and failures. It's great when the patient and practitioner line up and all runs smoothly, healing achieved. But that doesn't always happen. In terms of batting average, it probably doesn't even happen most of the time. The Three Pillars theory explains why.

Some might be put off by so many possibilities. But I write this to bring hope. I truly believe that there is an answer for almost all pain, even if it's not my answer.

That's an important thing for a medical practitioner to be able to say. We tend toward egotistical at times. We want to have all the answers, to heal all, to never disappoint a patient, to never disappoint ourselves. But it's critical, for our patients' sake, for us to remain humble and recognize our limits. We each have our strengths and specialties and we need to be willing to refer patients to others and admit when we cannot help.

≫ 15 ≪

The Well-Meaning
Mama Did It

"Her balance isn't so good. She has sensory processing issues," Diana urgently explained about her five-year-old daughter, Sarah. "Her legs are different lengths too. I have the same problem. Here," she continued, concerned, "I even brought her x-ray. See? One of her legs is clearly shorter than the other."

Usually, I received x-ray reports sent ahead of time. Diana carried Sarah's with her. This file was unusual, too, in that it was a full x-ray of both legs, from foot to pelvis.

I studied Sarah's image. Clearly her left hip was higher than her right.

"Yes, and is Sarah in pain?" I asked, a little confused.

"Not exactly," Diana said, "but look at her balance. It's hard for her to stand on one leg."

"Sarah, can you please stand on one leg for me?" I asked, turning to the fidgeting girl.

"Uh huh," she said as she stood on her left foot. She had to try several times before holding her balance on her leg for about 10 seconds.

"Can I see your other leg?" I asked.

"Sure," she said and stood on her right leg for about 30 seconds. She was much steadier.

"And watch her hop on one leg," Diana joined in. "Sarah, hop on one leg,"

Sarah hopped on her right leg. She landed in the same spot for about a minute.

"Now do your other one, dear," her mother said.

141

Sarah obediently hopped on the left leg. Sure enough, the foot landed in different places, like an amateur dart thrower trying to hit the bull's eye but only reaching the large outer ring of the board.

"Sarah," I said, "does it hurt to hop on your left leg?"

"Nope," she said, quickly glancing at her mother.

"I have the same thing," Diana said. "Ever since I was a girl, I've been accident prone and had weird aches and pains. Sarah has them too. She's just like Mama. Aren't you, sweetie?"

"Uh huh," Sarah nodded.

I studied Sarah's x-rays more closely. "So, Sarah's primary problem, as far as you can see, is that her balance is off, and she can't hop well on one leg?"

"And that one leg is longer. Yes, it's part of her sensory processing issues. We're seeing a specialist for them," Diana said with a worried look on her face.

"Well, I'm not well-versed on sensory processing issues, but if I could help Sarah with her hopping and balance, would you say that's what you've brought her here for?" I still wasn't clear about what the exact problem was, other than the leg length and balance issues.

"Yes, but you can't solve it. It's the way she's made. One leg is longer than the other. She needs shoe inserts to fix this. Hopefully that'll help her balance better and help her processing issues. I wear them too," she said.

"Oh, do you have a sensory processing issue as well?" I asked.

"Well, no one seems to know," she said. "But I think so."

"Okay, well, let me take a look at Sarah," I said, "and I'll see what I can do."

I evaluated Sarah and, sure enough, the left side of her pelvis was about an inch higher than her right. I showed her mother by putting my hands on the top of each side of Sarah's pelvis.

"So this is what you're talking about?" I turned to her.

"Exactly. That's why she needs shoe inserts. Just like Mama, right, Sarah?"

"I want to make sure you're seeing what I'm seeing," I replied to Diana. "Can you put your hands on top of Sarah's pelvis and confirm I'm seeing the right thing?"

I placed Diana's hands on the tops of Sarah's pelvis. "Now, kneel down so your eyes are at the level of her pelvis. That way you can see whether they're truly off."

Diana did as I asked. "I see it. You poor girl. We'll do our best honey, don't worry," she said.

I then asked Sarah to lie down on her back. "Sarah, I'm going to measure how long each of your legs are," I said. I grabbed my measuring tape from a nearby shelf and measured the length of her legs.

Practitioners measure the lengths of legs differently. Many measure them from a point on the pelvic bone down to the ankle bone or even the heel. If we measure from the pelvic bone to the ankle, that measurement crosses two joints: the hip joint and the knee joint. If we measure from the pelvis to the heel, that measurement includes three joints: the hip joint, knee joint and ankle joint.

It has long baffled me that some objective authority, a medical association, does not choose an optimal, universal way to measure. It would simplify matters to no end. I can imagine two reasons why it has not yet been done. First, medicine seems to proceed based on what's been done before. There are assumptions made early on that are never really challenged, so business carries on as usual until someone scratches their head and wonders about those precepts. You hear about this a few times a year, when a medical discovery turns our old ideas of how things work in the body on their head, paving the way for a more complete understanding of a phenomena. Second, leg length discrepancy is often something seen when standing and seeing one pelvis higher than the other. So naturally the pelvis should be included in the measurements. But I'd guess that this thinking occurred before anyone really understood how much a bone or joint rotates, contributing to the overall length of a limb. I've learned over the years that compensations occur through each joint in the chain which can contribute to the "appearance of a leg length discrepancy." After I realized how much the pelvic and ankle bones can be altered by muscle or ligament tightness or looseness, I realized I needed to take those out of the equation to get a true leg length measurement.

I've learned that the more joints you include in your measurement, the less reliable it becomes. This is because of subtle rotations that occur at each joint that make it appear that there are differences in length.

I measure from the top of the thigh bone to the ankle bone. This takes into account the length of the thigh and the lower leg bones and includes just one joint, the knee. The knee joint has less of a chance of rotation affecting the measurement.

Sarah's leg lengths were equal, according to my evaluation. She didn't have a leg length discrepancy. In my 20-plus years of measuring leg lengths in this way, I've perhaps come across just two or three patients who have more than a centimeter difference between their two legs. Yet I'd say 20 percent have been told by some medical practitioner that they have a leg length discrepancy.

I once gave a talk about this. A brave woman volunteered to come up for a demonstration. She told me she'd had a leg length discrepancy for years. I measured and found that her pelvis was uneven, but her legs were of equal length. I then corrected her pelvis, so it was level. Surprisingly, she wasn't happy with me. She'd had all her pants tailored to accommodate her uneven pelvis and would need to visit a tailor again—oops!

This confirmed to me that the differences in Sarah's apparent leg lengths were due to rotations at her joints. In Sarah's case, her left foot was flatter than her right, which would cause the left hip to drop down lower. Her left thigh muscles were tighter too. These attach to the front of the pelvic bone and rotate it forward, altering its appearance during measurements. Her left waist muscles tightened in an attempt to level her pelvis. They did too good a job at it. The left pelvis was held higher than the right by these muscles, similar to Sallie's case in Chapter 9.

I stretched Sarah's left thigh muscles, helped her left waist muscles release their spasm and taped up the arch of her left foot. I then measured her pelvic bones to see if they were level. They were.

"Diana, could you come over here and measure Sarah's pelvis for me? I just want to confirm what I'm seeing here," I said.

Diana came over, knelt down behind her daughter and measured the pelvic bones. "They're level," she said. "That's impossible. They can't be level. She has a difference in her leg lengths." She looked at me, perplexed. There was another emotion there I couldn't quite make out.

"Sarah doesn't have a leg length difference," I said, "Her foot is flatter on one side and a thigh muscle was tighter. This caused the

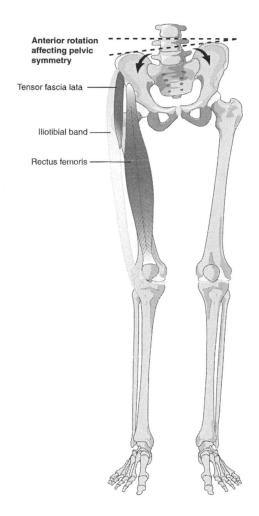

Anterior rotation
affecting pelvic
symmetry

Tensor fascia lata

Iliotibial band

Rectus femoris

A flat foot, together with tight thigh muscles, can make it appear as if a leg-length discrepancy exists.

waist muscles to lift that side of her pelvis, giving the appearance of a leg length discrepancy. My measurements show they are identical lengths. Sarah, can you please stand on your left foot?"

She did and stood for perhaps 20 seconds on that foot—definitely steadier than she'd been at the start of our session. This would improve even more if she practiced getting used to her level pelvis and having an arch that could help her.

"Sarah, can you hop around on your left foot?" I then asked.

Sarah dutifully hopped on her left foot. If the dart board distribution had been in the outer circle before, it was now in a much tighter formation, closer to the bull's eye. I then pulled out a miniature trampoline that we keep at the office.

"Sarah, can you hop on one leg on this little trampoline?" I asked.

This looked like fun, so she eagerly obliged, hopping first on her right foot for about 20 seconds.

"Now switch to your left foot, Sarah, if you would," I asked.

She then hopped on her left foot almost as well as her right. She was already learning from the improved alignment of her foot and pelvis.

Diana was flabbergasted and didn't seem all that pleased.

"How is this possible?!" she demanded. "She has a leg length discrepancy! She has x-rays to prove it!" She waved them in front of me.

"Well, it's true that it *looks* like she has a leg length discrepancy in the x-ray. But if you look closely, you can see that her left foot arch is slightly lower than the right. Now look at what that does to the ankle joint. Do you see how it's lined up differently than the right one? Look at the front of her lower leg bone. Do you see how it's pointing to the inside? Now look at the pelvic bone. See how that point is lower than the other side? These are all compensations occurring because of a flatter left foot and tighter thigh and waist muscles. We just corrected them, and she seems to be fine now. It's simple."

Diana became upset. I sensed that this might be her reaction, which is why I insisted that she measure Sarah's pelvis both times after I'd done so, so she wasn't just taking my word for it but saw it herself. She wasn't able to dispute the changes we made. Also, I made sure to have Sarah demonstrate her improved balance and coordination immediately after these changes, also so that her mother couldn't refute them.

You'd think that Diana would have been delighted. But a part of my job is psychology, not only helping people deal with problems but, occasionally, helping people digest good news when it goes against something they felt certain about. What I'd sensed from Diana's interactions up to this point was a need to validate her daughter's dysfunctions. I'm not sure why—that's for a full-time psychologist to weigh in on. Perhaps she was trying to validate her own problems by creating them in her daughter? Or perhaps she wanted her daughter to bond with her more closely by identifying so closely with her mother through a shared physical issue? There are many possible answers and working them out isn't my role, but it helps if I can sense them and ease the reception of news, whether that news is bad or good.

Whatever the reason, I felt it was my role to clearly show evidence that Sarah would be just fine—at least regarding the reasons Diana brought her into my clinic. There really was no leg length discrepancy and her balance improved significantly with just a couple of simple corrections.

I had not validated the story Diana was creating for her daughter. I showed her the truth of the matter. If Sarah was going to have a chance at a life in which her deficiencies weren't continually reinforced, then this was my opportunity to say no to that.

Diana and Sarah left and never returned.

Certainly, Diana was not intentionally trying to hurt her child. She was unaware of the psychological forces at work. Our beliefs and habits are deeply rooted in our experiences. We often pass those on to our children which can perpetuate that belief system. Patients will often say, "Well, I have a disc problem. My dad had it before me. My grandpa had before him. It's just how we're built."

Sometimes this is true. There may be some genetic issues behind this generational transmission of disc vulnerability, to give but one example. However, more likely it is an inherited belief system reinforced with learned behaviors, not an inherited physiological issue.

Children love to mimic their parents, especially when younger. They look up to them and want to be like them. They want their approval. I've seen them mimic their parents' walking patterns or gestures. They've learned how to walk (or bend or lift or run or work) the way their parents did.

But we need to consider someone's predisposition for a belief system too. For instance, my daughter was never interested in outdoor activities before our camping trip. She came with us to Minnesota and enjoyed herself, but not nearly as much as my son, who just loved every second.

Solving the Pain Puzzle

She will likely have a revulsion to camping or outdoor activities because of her one bad experience. She will reinforce this by not trying it again. If she goes on a hike, she might notice the unpleasant things—bugs, heat or fatigue—and ignore the pleasant aspects, like the view, breathing fresh air and exercising. Therefore, she'll never have an experience contrary to her one event. The absence of anything to the contrary reinforces beliefs. She is already building her belief system and shoring it up with examples.

It was important that I show Diana a definitive result that was contrary to the story she was developing for her daughter, and which, by extension, her daughter was adopting for herself. My hope was to interrupt their belief and behavior cycle. I tried to create a different set of experiences and expectations for them both.

Andrea and Beverley's stories in the previous two chapters showed how trauma and anxiety can become expressed as physical pain. Our beliefs contribute to our experience of pain too. Just look at people who walk across fire pits at corporate events for team building. They're taught in a day or two to believe they will not be hurt.

In Diana and Sarah's case, I saw what I felt were the building blocks of a belief system that would ultimately lead Sarah into thinking she was vulnerable, that she was not in control. These beliefs lead to a life of chronic pain. I couldn't let that happen to that little girl. I saw an opportunity to change her subconscious programming and perhaps steer them both to a different path of pain-free lives. I don't know how successful I was. From an objective perspective, I had "solved" the issue in a single session. It was really up to Diana, then, to decide that the truth was an acceptable new narrative. Otherwise, she could inadvertently hammer a weakness into her child who did not have one.

≋ 16 ≋

A Case Is Never
Truly Closed

By now you'll know that I love a good mystery. She walked into my clinic at 8 o'clock on a cool September morning. Little did I know that I would become obsessed with this woman's problem for the next two years and counting.

Sandra was an elegant 50-year-old woman with chronic debil-itating pain in the fourth and fifth fingers of her right hand. You might think that pain in these two fingers couldn't be *that* bad, after all, it's just her pinky and ring finger. We don't use those that often, do we? But Sandra described the pain as burning, stabbing, numbing, tingling, throbbing and sharp, rating the pain 10 out of 10. In med-icine, we reserve a 10 out of 10 rating for pain that results in emer-gency room visits. But from past experience, Sandra knew there was nothing an emergency room could do to help her. Her pain would last anywhere from minutes to hours. It would come and go and she couldn't predict when it would strike, filling her with dread through-out her day. Sandra worked at a computer and her pain would stop her in her tracks— she could focus on nothing else while it raged in her hand like a cornered wildcat. Years earlier, her problem put a halt to her five-days-a-week exercise program. At night she would drift in and out of sleep, the smallest random movement triggering this stab-bing pain that would last who knows how long.

As a teenager she'd played high school sports and had managed to escape without any serious injuries. Since then, she'd had breast implants 15 years before and had led a pain-free life with no other injuries or surgeries. Her pain gradually appeared more than 12 years before and worsened to the point where, after a plane flight, she would predictably have to sit doubled over and alone in the airport bathroom for 20 or more minutes waiting for it to subside. She didn't want anyone to see her in that condition. So she hid. The expansive possibilities of her life had constricted, squeezed by the pain. She was miserable. When she came to me, she said that her only hope to deaden the pain was through powerful medications which she hated to take, as they blunted her focus.

She also had swelling in her right hand, which had become slightly discolored as a result. This can happen when the arteries or veins are compromised, obstructing blood flow. Sandra's doctors concluded that she was suffering from thoracic outlet syndrome (TOS). The most common type of TOS involves squeezing all three nerves traveling down the arm and the blood vessels that accompany them too. That's why her hand was swollen—her blood circulation was impeded. The big squeeze usually happens somewhere between the neck bones and where the collarbone meets the shoulder. Symptoms of TOS typically involve pain in the shoulder area, forearm and/or hand and often cold or weakness in the hand.

In Sandra's case, pain in the fourth and fifth fingers indicated a problem with the ulnar nerve that feeds them. The nerves to the hand originate from the lower levels of the neck (C5-T1). There is one nerve exiting each spinal level. These then merge to form the brachial plexus, an area where they cross and combine like a bird's eye view of a particularly busy section of a Los Angeles overpass, finally distilling down to three larger nerves, the journeys of which end in the hand.

Think of the hand like a mountain lake into which three rivers flow. Each of those rivers carries water from five different peaks of the surrounding mountains. The three nerves feeding our hand are the ulnar, median and radial nerves, and each feeds a different part of the hand. The ulnar nerve only receives water from two of the peaks, C8 and T1.

These nerves have established pathways. They must contend with structures around which they wrap, under which they duck or through which they pierce—it's like a nerve obstacle course. It can be a perilous journey for those thin little guys getting messages to and from the hand to the neck and ultimately the spinal cord.

The ulnar nerve is no exception in this regard. Much like an action movie hero, the ulnar nerve valiantly carries his secret messages across hostile territory all day long without anyone suspecting his mission or paying attention to him—until he's hurt.

Its first hurdle is just getting clear of the neck bones which can become arthritic or shift to compress the nerve roots. Next, our little messenger travels through neck muscles (the scalenes), the grip of which can lock him in a chokehold. Then it passes between the collarbone and our first rib, a low cave he must shimmy through on his stomach before diving underneath a small chest muscle (the pectoralis minor) that could mash it into the rib cage like a WWF smackdown. At this point, our ulnar nerve has been accompanied by his brother and sister, the median and radial nerves, as well as blood vessels feeding the arm. But from here on, he becomes a lone hero to finish his job.

Our poor little ulnar nerve, alone but determined, runs down the inner part of the upper arm where, just like a bed sheet that's too tight, it can be bound by a layer of fascia. Our messenger then finds himself in a bony tunnel (the tarsal tunnel) at the elbow. If the ulnar nerve were flying on Elbow Airlines, he would always have a center seat on the plane. In a perfect world, our little guy would be sitting between two supermodels, so he would have plenty of room to move around and be happy. Sometimes, though, the bones of the tarsal tunnel thicken and his seatmates, now the size of NFL linemen, squeeze him unmercifully to the point where he can't even wiggle in his seat. That's what tarsal tunnel syndrome is like and it's no wonder that it could be responsible for Sandra's pain.

After he clears the elbow, our ulnar nerve hero happily runs down the inner forearm, before continuing across the wrist bones which, just in case he thought he was home free, could shift or fracture, wounding him.

If Sandra decided to rest on her palm a little too long in one position, she could inadvertently crush her ulnar nerve in its final leg of his journey to feed the fourth and fifth fingers.

I suffered an ulnar nerve crush injury by leaning on my hand over the course of three days while I varnished my front porch with a hand brush. Not an action that you'd expect would lead to injury! A typical ulnar nerve crush injury isn't painful: the fourth and fifth fingers simply become very weak. I had to stop playing guitar for months while the nerve regrew and strength returned. I now use a roller brush to varnish my front porch—not only does it protect my ulnar nerve but I'm done in an hour or two!

Thankfully, doctors can perform something called a "nerve conduction velocity test" to determine if the nerve is obstructed at any of these obstacles. Sandra had this done and it came back showing some minor obstruction, yes, but no definite points were evident.

Interestingly, through the course of her tests and images (x-rays and the like), the doctors found she had an extra rib in her neck. This is called a "cervical rib." Cervical ribs are found in about 1 percent of healthy people and about 30 percent of those diagnosed with TOS. She not only had one but two, one on each side of her neck, which is even more rare. A cervical rib is really just a nub of a rib—not like other ribs. But the presence of this "riblet" throws a monkey wrench into the whole brachial plexus machine. It tends to crowd an already busy area. That crowding can affect the nerves and blood vessels feeding the arm.

By the time Sandra arrived at my office for the first time, she'd had surgeries to shave those NFL linemen in her elbow down to size so her ulnar nerve had some more (pardon the pun but I just can't resist) elbow room. Her doctors also removed part of her first rib, to drop the floor of the cave at the collarbone, giving the nerve more room to scoot through. They also removed the cervical rib on that side of her neck and had one of her scalene muscles severed, to release the chokehold on the nerves passing through.

These last three surgeries solved one problem, the swelling and coldness in her right hand. But to everyone's surprise, none of them helped her hand pain. So, in exasperation, her doctor sent her my way.

I conducted her initial evaluation as gently as possible and found several potential suspects. I have a unique approach to helping people with TOS and thought this would be a slam dunk. But when she reported that her pain was much worse *after* our first session, I knew I had something different on my hands. I've worked with enough people with TOS or it's cousin, carpal tunnel syndrome, to know what to expect. Sandra didn't behave anything like these patients.

I was immediately suspicious—something unusual was going on here.

For her next visit, I decided to explore her forearm, since her symptoms only involved her hand and, occasionally, her forearm—perhaps the issue was lower down than anyone else had been looking? I gently massaged those muscles, paying particular attention to the pathway of the ulnar nerve. I was feeling for knots or restrictions that might trigger her hand pain but found none.

Sandra returned later in the week, reporting that her symptoms were much worse *after* our massage. Unfortunately, this became a common refrain in our work together as I tried to unravel her mystery.

Each visit I would focus on a different area to flush out our culprit. I explored her upper arm, then her shoulder blade, armpit, chest muscles, upper back muscles, and her neck. All my attempts over the course of several weeks resulted not only in no solution but in more pain for her. The Hippocratic Oath states, "First, do no harm." And here I was, with the best of intentions, but making my patient feel worse after each session than she had before.

I felt terrible—I couldn't remember the last time I had failed so thoroughly. All my go-to tricks had failed. Why was she even sticking with me?

Finally, I found a group of muscles that would give her the slightest bit of relief—the serratus anterior muscles.

The serratus anterior muscles are a funky group that begin along various levels of the upper and middle rib cage in the front and attach to the shoulder blade in the back. They lie along the side of the rib cage in the armpit area. Lightly massaging here would give her relief for perhaps a day, maybe two.

That's as far as we got. After several weeks of this, we both realized that this ultimately wasn't going to solve her problem.

She drifted off my schedule, while I guided her through various doctor appointments, testing other theories of potential sources of irritation. If my own sessions weren't leading to a definitive improvement, I wanted to at least assist her with finding another medical professional who might help.

One possibility was that her breast implant could have leaked, irritating the chest muscles, which was one of my discoveries during our initial exam. That turned out to be another dead end—her implants were intact. Then a cortisone shot to her pectoralis minor—the only muscle that wasn't operated on for her TOS. I pinned a lot of my hopes on this procedure. But, again, it failed.

What was I missing? My mind drifted to my visit about 10 years earlier to Regis University's cadaver lab to brush up on my anatomy. During my years as a PT, I grew to appreciate the uniqueness of each body I worked with, while also keeping in mind the general rules of the game. So, aside from my specific questions I came there to answer (why the shoulder was important to trigeminal neuralgia, what I was affecting when I mobilized the shoulder blade the way I did to create change), I slowly lingered over each cadaver, noting differences in muscle thickness, areas of muscle insertions, differences in bony architecture of the pelvis and shoulder blades, the lengths of Achilles tendons, the thickness of foot fat pads, the movement of hip joints in a cadaver with anteverted femurs versus retroverted femurs and how the joint capsule that surrounds the socket twists and untwists based on these differences, the relative thickness of people's suboccipital muscles at the base of their skulls and their insertions into the neck bones or the proximity of these insertions to the levator scapula—that muscle from the shoulder blade that causes so much pain.

No two were alike, of course, but I was thinking of these differences as they related to pain. How would this person's neck respond to my manual techniques if I were to perform a suboccipital release? I performed releases on the cadavers and noted exactly where my fingers were coming into contact with their necks or skulls. What tissues are taken up first if I were to add distraction to the equation?

I carried a notebook with me, which ended up being a bunch of scribbles even I had a difficult time decoding once I returned home. Textbooks make it seem like we're all built the same, with clearly defined borders of muscles, ligaments and bones—exploring a range of cadavers makes it clear that this is not so.

I learned there that I needed to be more patient with my patients and myself. I learned to keep in mind this variety when working with people, to be willing to experiment to accommodate their unique architecture with a slight rotation here or a gentle mobilization there to create the changes I thought were needed.

As I traced these variations, I began to speculate why one person might be good at an activity, say tennis, as opposed to someone else. Further, it appeared that the deeper, smaller muscles were

154

more diverse than the larger, more superficial muscles. I'm sure this was pointed out when I was a student, but it was lost on me because I was too concerned at the time with memorizing the origin, insertion, innervation and action of the muscles—not their variability. I pondered their roles in stabilization and power generation. I wished, at that moment, that I could have sat down with each cadaver, have had a conversation about their life and watched them move, to test my ideas.

I received many valuable insights during that visit. Each person is unique, and medical practitioners would do well to remember that more often than we do. The presence of Sandra's cervical ribs was yet more evidence. What if Sandra had some type of anomaly that I'd never heard of? After all, this is the human body we're talking about. This potential variant would need to occur after the ulnar nerve separated from the rest of his family, the median and radial nerves, as well as the blood vessels. That would put it somewhere around the pectoralis minor muscle, deep in the chest near the armpit. But I'd explored these possibilities already. Where could it be? Had I missed something?

I searched for two hours on the Internet and found an interesting anomaly I'd never heard of before—an axillary arch. Axillary is the fancy word for "armpit." This is an extra portion of a big flaring muscle you see in body builders that gives them their trademark V shape—the latissimus dorsi, "lats" for short.

This muscle can shoot off a little extra runner, like a strawberry plant looking for new places to grow. That runner attaches further up the arm, closer to the armpit. The nerves traveling down the arm pass right through that arch which can constrict them. It's rare, occurring in about 7 percent of the population. That's enough of an anomaly that most doctors have never even heard of it. This means that radiologists who read MRIs also might miss it because they're not looking for it.

After further research, I found that a little runner can also emerge from our big chest muscle, the pectoralis major, our "pecs." Similar to the lats, the pecs send off a little slip of muscle, called the chondroepitrochlearis, to attach on the upper portion of the arm. This, likewise, forms an arch and can trap nerves or blood vessels.

I referred Sandra to a shoulder surgeon for a cortisone shot and an MRI. I hoped, like Justin (the big linebacker with neck pain), the cortisone shot would clear her pain temporarily and, in so doing, show that something was wrong in her shoulder joint. But she had no relief from her shot. I knew this was a long shot since my treatment hadn't picked up the shoulder as a culprit but I thought it was worth a try anyway. At least this let me rule out her shoulder joint as the problem.

We waited two weeks for her MRI appointment. In the meantime, I called the radiologist to inform him that I suspected an axillary arch or pectoral arch as the culprit. He hadn't heard of either of these anomalies, so I sent him some research articles. He promised he'd try to find them.

I was excited because these variations apparently cause neurological pain in at least 70 percent of the people who have them. I was running out of ideas for Sandra and needed to solve this mystery. This was the best lead yet.

I received Sandra's shoulder/armpit MRI report: negative. I felt like I'd been punched in the gut. The two arches seemed like the perfect solution. Additionally, she had another MRI of her brachial plexus region—where all the nerve and bone traffic congests near the neck. Negative. I was shut down at every turn.

I decided to go for gold and contact the author of one of the papers I'd found on the pectoral arch. He was a peripheral nerve specialist at a prestigious medical center, a specialist in nerves after they exit the spinal cord. I hoped I could pique his interest with a difficult case. Sandra said she was open to flying out to see him if he was interested. He responded that he had nothing to offer.

I could only think of one more test to order: a guided dynamic ultrasound. The benefit of this test is that the patient can move their body while the tester uses an ultrasound to "see" what tissues might be damaged or impinged during those movements. This is an especially good choice for someone who has intermittent pain or pain with a particular movement and whose MRI showed no problems. It seemed perfect for Sandra's case. I contacted Sandra's primary care doctor, who by this time was probably getting tired of all my special requests, to order one for her. My goal was to target the armpit and chest muscles, as well as to revisit the elbow tunnel, to see if something had been missed there.

Again, I contacted the radiologist prior to testing. He was part of a special group focused on more difficult cases. They were not familiar with either of the variants I was looking for and I sent them the research articles I'd uncovered. I'd even found one article describing the technique they used to "see" the chondroepitrochlearis they were looking for. This described the patient's arm position and had the patient exert some effort to cause the targeted muscle to contract, thereby showing up on the ultrasound better. I highlighted this for the radiologist and discussed the arm positioning and muscular contraction pattern we needed to achieve, in order to visualize either the axillary arch or its cousin from the chest muscle. He was very kind to listen to me and became excited at the prospect of looking for these variants if they existed, as he had not had a case like this before. My fingers were crossed. I finally had someone on my side interested in Sandra's case.

Unfortunately, all testing was put on hold due to the coronavirus. Sandra and I had to wait it out. While waiting, I continued to sift through her signs and symptoms. I found myself doubting her test results. Did the breast implant doctor really look well enough? Did the radiologist really get the image he needed to see these anomalies, and could he decipher one if he did, never having seen one before?

Eventually the testing was completed—no variants detected. All the wind was again knocked out of my sails. I can't imagine what Sandra must've been feeling at this news. So many dead ends, and I was the one leading her to most of them. I wouldn't have blamed her if she hadn't wanted to hear from me again.

Several months passed and I had no other leads. About this time, I had been helping one of my therapists with a shoulder problem. Finally, we decided she needed some imaging. She had a unique pattern of pain, and we thought that a dynamic ultrasound would be the best option.

She found a doctor to do it. It came back that she had a biceps tear. But she was really impressed with her doctor. He spoke excitedly about her shoulder and his work and had mentioned that he'd recently discovered a phenomenon in which the shoulder can leak fluid, irritating adjacent structures, including nerves. Neither of us had heard of this and I think he was having a hard time getting other doctors to listen. This sounded like a doctor who was willing to experiment and investigate unusual issues. My lightbulb went on. Could this be the doctor we needed for Sandra?

I got her on the phone and explained this new phenomenon to her. She agreed to see him for another dynamic ultrasound. I also wrote up a synopsis of her case, including surgeries, tests and conclusions. His office had never received this type of information from a physical therapist before—I'm not sure how they took it. Nevertheless, they agreed to look for the variants, as well as the possibility of a leaking shoulder joint. Sandra and I once again were very excited about the results.

But, once again, all tested negative.

The doctor traced out the entire ulnar nerve during the testing, from hand to neck, and found nothing wrong. He gave her a cortisone shot in her wrist to shrink tissues potentially impinging the ulnar nerve there.

Again, no change in her symptoms. I was baffled.

Soon after this, Sandra saw another doctor who injected three levels of vertebrae in her neck, her deeper chest muscle that could potentially trap the ulnar nerve (the pectoralis minor) and her forearm muscles. Once again, no change in her symptoms. She was fed up with all the testing and injections. I felt we had turned over every stone I and every other doctor could think of.

But there is never no answer. Walls are meant to be climbed. So many highly intelligent medical professionals with decades of experience between them trying to figure this out. So many tests. So many surgeries. All to no avail. What could it mean?

It meant I was looking in the wrong places. But what other places could there be?

I thought about all of this for weeks. I needed to shift my point of view. Then it struck me that we all were looking at the ulnar nerve pathway from a musculoskeletal perspective, as I described at the beginning of the chapter. The nerve had a certain obstacle course it must traverse to get to the hand. But what if there were another adjacent obstacle that wasn't part of the course, influencing the others?

I went back to my initial evaluation. One finding that never added up for me was her tender right chest muscle. That didn't fit with her complaints, because the larger chest muscle doesn't interact with the ulnar nerve. I'd put it aside to pursue more obvious solutions.

Not being an expert in breast augmentation complications, I assumed the only thing that could irritate that chest muscle was a leaking implant. We had pursued that idea and cleared it early on in our attempts to help her. But what if there were other issues of which I wasn't aware?

Once again, I went back to research for complications from breast implants. Most articles dealt with shoulder or chest pain as a result. Some indicated TOS complaints that resolved with surgery. Sandra had already had surgery for TOS which helped some symptoms but not this remaining painful symptom. Then I found one lonely blog article that described intermittent ulnar nerve pain that had stumped practitioners.

I discovered a phenomenon called "capsular contracture," where the breast implant hardens and scar tissue develops, constricting the capsule around the breast implant. This becomes like another hard surface pushing up against the TOS region of the neck and shoulder. This might explain why her right chest muscle was so tender. After all, this occurred three years *after* her implant surgery. That may be the amount of time it took for her body to build scar tissue enough to impinge upon nearby structures.

When I asked her to have her implant checked for leakage a year earlier, she told her doctor about her ulnar nerve pain and TOS issues. However, the doctor apparently assumed they were unrelated.

I called Sandra to talk about this possibility. It was only a few days after her last series of injections to multiple sites that bore no fruit. She was tired and fed up. This time I didn't hear the cheerful woman I'd been working with for two years. Instead, she sounded wary, doubtful and mistrusting of me.

"Maybe I just have to put up with it," she said.

"Sandra, I know I've said this before and you've no reason to believe me, but we've cleared everything that could be affecting the ulnar nerve. This has to be it! Hang in there just a little longer!" I urged.

I didn't want her to give up. I saw our past failures as clues to the real culprit—kind of like putting culprits in jail for a crime spree only to find the same crimes keep happening. They must not be the right culprits.

Now that we'd approached every possibility, we had to consider a new set of offenders. Maybe her sore chest muscle just a few years after her implant surgery was more than just a coincidence. It was a clue we'd all been ignoring but couldn't any longer.

As I sit here at my kitchen table writing this, I can barely contain myself. I haven't even had a cup of coffee, but I'm wired, buzzing with anticipation. This might be the answer, finally. This is a case I'm writing about in the middle of the action, not in retrospect. It's a thriller of a medical mystery for which I don't yet know the answer.

If this ends up being the source of her pain, how would this explain her most consistent irritant—traveling on a plane? It only takes a brief imaginary visit to your run-of-the-mill tight quarters on an airplane to come up with a theory. The seats are never wide enough, and throughout the flight, especially if you haven't won the battle for using the arm rest, your shoulder and chest must subtly work with the effort of holding your arm toward your body throughout the flight. If she had a contracture in her chest area, this would likely heighten it, thereby pressing the hardened tissue more firmly into the ulnar nerve space, compressing it ever so slightly. Sandra's report of her pain was that it occurred intermittently without any particular pattern. If we consider my three pillars of pain theory, this means that she must be very close to her pain threshold at all times. Any slight provocation will push her through the threshold. This is what prolonged chest contraction would do to her, such as trying not to touch the person sitting too close to her on a flight.

I asked her to return to her surgeon to explore this possibility. I'm waiting on pins and needles. Her story, as I complete this book, has not been fully resolved, which is difficult for me to accept. I still hold out hope that, prior to this publication, we will find her answer. While it seems strange to include an unfinished story in my book, it is also fitting. It illustrates the struggles that some people, and practitioners, have to find solutions. I see this as blessing and a curse of the miracle of our existence. The seemingly infinite permutations of form, function and response to some adverse element fascinates me. And this is only the musculoskeletal system. Thanks to this, I'm always kept on my toes.

><

As a postscript to this chapter, Sandra's doctor confirmed there are no complications from her implants. I still haven't given up on her, though...

I hope that this book has expanded your understanding of your anatomy and pain. My greatest hope is that, if you are one of those who have been searching for answers to your pain, these stories perhaps offer a glimpse into new possibilities to solve your issue. I wish you success.

Index

Numbers in *bold italics* indicate pages with illustrations